Continuity and Adaptation in Aging

Continuity and Adaptation in Aging

Creating Positive Experiences

Robert C. Atchley

The Johns Hopkins University Press

Baltimore and London

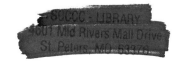

© 1999 The Johns Hopkins University Press
All rights reserved. Published 1999
Printed in the United States of America on acid-free paper
9 8 7 6 5 4 3 2 1

The Johns Hopkins University Press
2715 North Charles Street
Baltimore, Maryland 21218-4363
www.press.jhu.edu

ISBN 0-8018-6122-5

| Contents

Preface   *vii*
Acknowledgments   *xv*

1 Continuity Theory   1

   How Did Continuity Theory Arise?   1
   Continuity Theory as Theory   4
   Elements of Continuity Theory   9
   Development versus Aging in Later Adulthood   12
   Case Examples   13

2 Internal Continuity   33

   Continuity of the Self   34
   Self-Confidence   35
   Emotional Resilience   41
   Personal Goals   44
   Beliefs about the Effects of Retirement   47
   Summary   51

3 External Continuity   53

   Living Arrangements, Household Composition, and
      Marital Status   54
   Income Adequacy   56
   Modes of Transportation   57
   Patterns of Activity: Stability, Continuity, and
      Change over Time   57
   How Activities Fit Together to Form Lifestyles   70
   Summary   74

4 Adaptive Capacity 76

Proactive Coping and Motivation for Continuity 78
How Did Respondents Cope? 82
Coping with Specific Changes: Retirement, Widowhood,
    and Functional Limitations 85
Functional Limitation and the Self 93
Patterns of Coping with Functional Limitations 107
General Patterns of Adaptation 118
Factors Linked to Negative Outcomes in Later Life 126
Summary 130

5 Goals for Developmental Direction 133

Continuity of Personal Goals 133
Disposition toward Continuity 136
Spiritual Development 139
The Theory of Gerotranscendence 142
The Study of Goals for Developmental Direction in
    Later Life 145

6 Conclusion 147

Assessing Continuity Theory 148
Evidence on the Assumptions and Propositions of
    Continuity Theory 150
Continuity Strategies Are Generally Effective 154
Methodological Issues Related to the Study of
    Continuity Theory 155
Future Research Using Continuity Theory 156

Appendixes
A. Tables 159
B. The Ohio Longitudinal Study of Aging and Adaptation 161
C. The 1995 Study Questionnaire 172
D. Worksheets Used to Examine Longitudinal Patterns 197

References 203
Index 209

| *Preface*

    This book is about how people evolve psychologically and socially as they age and adapt to change. Continuity theory holds that adult development and adaptation are continuous. This theory was created to explain the common empirical finding that a large majority of aging adults manage to maintain physical, psychological, and social well-being and satisfying relationships and lifestyles in a society that is youth oriented and often antagonistic toward aging and older people. Continuity theory presumes that most people learn continuously from their life experiences and intentionally continue to grow and evolve in directions of their own choosing. Continuity theory is a general theory that attempts to explain why continuity of ideas and lifestyles is central to the process of adult development in midlife and later and why continuity is such a common strategy for coping with changes in middle and later life.

    Gerontology has often been described as atheoretical, perhaps because its journals are filled with research reports that are best described as abstracted empiricism, loaded with description and statements of relation tied to operational measures rather than to interconnected theoretical constructs that constitute full-fledged theory. Despite this common misperception, gerontology actually has many theories just on individual aging, and these theories cover a wide variety of topics: the stages of adult development (Erikson et al. 1986; Levinson 1990), stress and coping in later life (Skaff 1995; Pearlin 1991), the stresses of caregiving (Kinney et al. 1995; Biegel and Blum 1990), social isolation in old age (Kuypers and Bengtson 1973; Bennett 1980), adaptation to role loss (Cumming and Henry 1961; Havighurst 1963; Rosow 1967; Lemon et al. 1972; Longino and Kart 1982; Atchley 1985), and the life course (Atchley 1975a; Hagestad 1990), just to name a few. Dozens of plausible theories are buried in the literature of gerontology, yet none has captured the imaginations of gerontologists sufficiently to become an organizing framework for the significant streams of thought or research necessary to become a recognized general theory of individual development and adaptation to aging. Continuity theory was created in the hope of meeting this need — no modest task.

To advance theory we cannot merely present general descriptions and conceptual frameworks, necessary and useful as these may be. We must also show how theoretical frameworks can be used in research and how theories relate to actual human lives. Three major goals of this book are to elaborate continuity theory, to show how it can be used, and to test some of its major tenets empirically.

The data used to work with continuity theory come from a study that for 20 years followed more than a thousand individuals who were age 50 or older in 1975. By 1995, there were more than 300 people still participating in the study. At periodic intervals between 1975 and 1995, the participants filled out questionnaires aimed at documenting their inner psychological frameworks of beliefs, attitudes, values, goals, motives, emotions, and temperament, as well as the external social frameworks that made up their lifestyles: household composition, marital status, number of children, occupation, employment status, leisure activities, involvement in community organizations, and involvement with family and friends. Respondents also provided background information such as race, gender, age, religious affiliation, and education. Many questions concerned health and disability over the course of the study because we were especially interested in how people adapted to changes in health. Other questions dealt with retirement and widowhood because these are major role changes that usually occur after 50. Finally, many questions dealt with financial resources, especially income adequacy and sources of retirement income.

For all aspects of adult development, aging, and adaptation considered in this book, there were both positive and negative changes over time among the study participants. Development was often a growth process, and although physical and psychological aging generally produced modest declines with age, there were respondents whose physical health and psychological outlook improved over time as they grew older. The consequences of social aging for lifestyles were generally minor. An overwhelming majority of the study participants were able to adapt well to the changes they experienced over the 20 years of the study.

This book uses these longitudinal data to identify areas of continuity and areas of stability as well as to chart the various ways in which the study participants experienced discontinuity. It also looks at how people adapted to various types of change, ranging from gradual and minor physical changes to profound disability, from minor swings in morale and motivation to a sharp downturn in mood, from minor shifts in social roles to complete disengagement from some social roles, from minor changes in social support networks to sharp reductions in the size of social networks.

Background

For more than 30 years I have been interested in how people adapt to the changes associated with aging. I began my research in gerontology in 1963, with a study of how retirement influenced the self-concepts of retired women. At that time gerontology was involved intensely in the controversy sparked by the disengagement theory of Elaine Cumming and William Henry (1961), which proclaimed that both psychological and social disengagement were mutually desired and beneficial for individual elders and for society as well. This theory was opposed vigorously by activity theory (Havighurst 1963; Rosow 1967), which held that elders adjust best by finding replacements for lost activities or relationships and by maintaining activity at a level comparable to that in middle age. Both of these theories addressed the causes and consequences of role loss in later life, and both were taken as theories of how to adapt successfully to aging.

As I began my dissertation on the impact of retirement on women's self-concepts and self-esteem, I developed a series of hypotheses that predicted negative effects for the self when women retired and thus no longer had a work identity. But as I was pretesting my interview schedule, I was brought up short by a woman who, at the end of a pretest interview, said, "Is that it? When are you going to ask me about the good stuff about retirement?" I realized that I had unconsciously biased the interview by asking only about areas where negative effects of retirement might be expected. Using focus groups of retired women, I developed a more balanced set of questions.

I was thoroughly impressed with the positive adjustment I found among both retired women schoolteachers and retired women telephone operators. By and large, they had strong and resilient self-concepts, high self-esteem, and a firm sense of values that informed their everyday decision making. Of course, both of these occupational groups had adequate retirement pensions even before major changes increased the generosity of Social Security benefits in 1972. None of the negative effects I expected materialized because these women carried their occupational identities with them into retirement and continued to derive self-esteem from them (Atchley 1967, 1976a).

In 1968, I conducted a similar study with a sample of more than 4,000 retired teachers and telephone company employees of both genders and again found that an overwhelming majority were well adjusted to retirement, had carried over occupational identities, and had high self-esteem (Atchley 1971a, 1971b). Men and women adapted to retirement equally well, although there were substantial other gender differences (Atchley 1976b).

The observation that most people carried their occupational identity over into retirement and thus maintained their identity led to a preliminary statement of a theory of identity continuity (Atchley 1971a) in opposition to the still-popular identity crisis theory. Identity continuity theory stated simply that elders have a large amount of evidence from the past upon which they can rest their claim to an occupational identity even though they may no longer be engaged in that occupation for pay. Identity crisis theory (Miller 1965) posited that no longer playing occupational roles would inevitably precipitate an identity crisis in a work-oriented society such as ours. However, identity crisis theory has never fit more than a very small proportion of the cases in the five different studies of retirement adaptation that I conducted over a span of 20 years, nor does it fit the major findings of a large majority of the studies of retirement that are based on representative populations (Atchley 1982a; Parnes 1985; Ekerdt 1995).

Although in my studies only a very small minority of people experienced social withdrawal, declining morale, or declining physical health as a result of retirement, anecdotal and clinical reports still stress negative outcomes of retirement. I continued to be curious about the mechanisms that might cause people to have difficulty adapting to retirement. I thought it possible that external social circumstances such as age discrimination in the labor market for those who wished to work part time in retirement might lead to negative effects on the self and on life satisfaction. I also thought it possible that people might become disenchanted with retirement if their preretirement plans turned out to be unrealistic (Atchley 1976c, 1979).

Most research on retirement adaptation published before 1975 was cross-sectional. Researchers compared retirees with people of similar age who remained employed, and the differences were attributed to retirement, or retirees were asked to look back retrospectively and compare their situation in retirement with their situation just before retirement. Many articles on retirement adaptation called for longitudinal studies that would follow the same people as they went through the retirement transition. I began the Ohio Longitudinal Study of Aging and Adaptation (OLSAA) in 1975 to fill some of these gaps. (For a more detailed description of the study, see the appendixes.) During that time, several other longitudinal studies of retirement were begun, including the National Longitudinal Studies of the Labor Market Experiences of Mature Men (Parnes 1985) and the Normative Aging Study (Bossé and Spiro 1995). Both of these studies were much more ambitious than the OLSAA, but they included only men.

Funded initially by a seven-year grant from the National Institute of Mental Health and later by the Ohio Long-Term Care Research Project, the OLSAA was designed to survey the entire population who were age 50 or older and residents of a small town in middle America as of July 1, 1975. The goal was to survey the panel at two-year intervals and document their adaptation to aging and retirement.

The town represents an ideal environment for retirement in many respects. It is near a large city, it is a college town with many opportunities for activity, it has a full range of health and social service programs, and it has remained relatively free of urban problems such as crime and neighborhood blight. The target population was surveyed in 1975, 1977, 1979, and 1981. Then funding for the study ceased. However, in 1990 additional funding was secured from the Ohio Long-Term Care Research Project, and the panel was surveyed again in 1991 and 1995. The number of respondents over the six waves of the study was 1,106, 852, 678, 667, 474, and 335. Response rates for the surveys were 75 percent or higher. By 1995, all of the remaining panel members were age 70 or older. Of the original panel, 347 had died, 260 had dropped out, and 332 had moved or were lost to follow-up. (For a discussion of the implications of attrition in the study population, see the appendixes.)

Before the OLSAA, my research on adaptation had concentrated mainly on the relationship between self and role, but I began to see the need for a broader perspective. My thinking was influenced by the integration of several disparate but complementary perspectives. In the late 1960s, I came to appreciate feedback systems theory (Buckley 1967) as a type of theory with tremendous potential for understanding the ongoing evolution of an individual's social psychological framework of ideas. Buckley's feedback systems theory assigned great importance to life experience in the evolution of a person's ideas about what is true and what works in the world. I also felt that looking ahead played a significant role in adaptation. I hypothesized that the existence of idealized life course norms produced a degree of predictability that for most people prevented most life course events from becoming crises in identity, morale, health, or lifestyle (Atchley 1975a). At the conference where I presented this life course paper, Klaus Riegel presented his dialectical theory of continuous adult development (Riegel 1976), which focused on the continuous, contingent, and emergent influence of contradictions and paradoxes on everyday adult development. This perspective invited us to reconsider the prominent stage theories of adult development, especially Erikson's cumulative stage theory (Erikson 1963). In the early 1980s, I learned about George Kelly's (1955) personal construct theory, which was my first exposure to constructivist thought. The idea that individuals developed their own unique interpretations of the world "out there," were active agents in the production of their own subjective realities, and based their actions on their resulting personal constructs fit very well the data I had collected on identity continuity.

As I was absorbing and integrating these various theoretical strands, I was also analyzing data from the initial waves of the OLSAA. By 1981 it was clear that retirement had little or no effect on a person's degree of adaptation, however measured (1982b). Disability, on the other hand, had moderate negative effects on activity level and self-confidence. Accordingly, I included more questions about disability on each successive wave of the OLSAA questionnaires, beginning in 1979.

My first attempt at a complete statement of continuity theory was published in 1989 (Atchley 1989). From 1989 to 1995, more than 25 studies referred to continuity theory as an orienting framework. From 1993 to 1997, I published several papers that refined and tested aspects of continuity theory and developed methods for measuring continuity and differentiating it from both absolute stability and discontinuity (Atchley 1993, 1995, 1996, 1997a, 1997b).

In many ways, this book takes readers on a tour of adult development and adaptation in later adulthood that took me more than 30 years to map. I developed this map from studying people age 50 or older, not by extending theories of child development. I developed it by a combination of quantitative and qualitative methods, not just from clinical observations, or mail questionnaires, or structured interviews but also from observations of elders in a variety of formal and informal settings and in-depth, open-ended interviews. The map is still crude in many places, but I believe that the results show that continuity theory consists of a body of concepts, causal relationships, and research methods that can be very helpful as we try to understand the later-life development of the upcoming generations of elders.

The Plan of the Book

To evaluate continuity theory we must first be clear about what we mean by continuity, how and where we can look for evidence of it, and the multidimensional nature of it. We can then lay out various concepts and theoretical propositions of continuity theory and examine the various elements of the theory in terms of how well the data fit.

This book is organized as follows: Chapter 1 describes the development of continuity theory, presents the various elements of the theory in detail, and discusses the methodological issues involved in studying it. Chapter 1 closes with case examples that illustrate the difference between continuity and discontinuity. Chapter 2 looks at evidence for continuity in patterns of thought such as the self-concept, self-confidence, and personal goals. Chapter 3 examines evidence for continuity over time in the external social arrangements that make up lifestyle, including household composition, living arrangements, and lifestyle activities. Chapter 4 is the most complex chapter. It looks at how continuity relates to adaptation, coping, and adaptive capacity. It also considers motivation for adaptation and proactive coping, various types of coping, and how study participants coped with specific changes such as retirement, widowhood, and the onset of physical disability. Chapter 4 ends with case histories showing the relation between continuity and adaptation to aging and various life changes associated with aging. Chapter 5 deals with goals for developmental direction, which provide motivation to orient change in directions that support continuity. The chapter considers continuity of personal goals over time, disposition toward continuity, and goals for spiritual development, which may become more important in later adulthood. Chapter 6 starts with a general review of the findings in relation to continuity theory. It then considers some negative aspects of continuity as an adaptive strategy, methodological issues related to the study of continuity, and some ideas concerning future research on continuity theory.

Gender and social class are important social structural variables that are used very early in life by various gatekeepers to determine people's access to education and occupational roles. Gender and social class also influence access to community roles and modify both personal and social performance expectations in a variety of roles. Women and people of lower social class are generally at a disadvantage in terms of access to education, higher occupational levels, and community leadership. There has been some improvement in the status of women over the past 30 years, but most women are still concentrated in jobs that have traditionally been defined as "women's work," and this is particularly true for the cohorts of women in this study. Accordingly, in each chapter we consider gender and social class differences within the context of the chapter's theme.

| *Acknowledgments*

It is usual in the preface to give thanks where thanks are due. The statement "Show me a person with a new idea and I'll show you a person with a poor memory" seems to apply well to me. The only thing novel about my approach to adult development is its unique combination of already existing ideas. I have learned so much from so many people that it would literally be impossible to thank them all. Most of them are cited in the references to this book, but ideas grow and get connected to other ideas through a process of integration that benefits a great deal from feedback. I especially appreciate being able to discuss continuity theory and my research on adult development with Fred Cottrell, Millie Seltzer, Lillian Troll, Sheila Atchley, Dale Dannefer, Carol Ryff, Victor Marshall, and Suzanne Kunkel. I probably learned the most from the challenges that these friends posed and the gaps they identified, although it is always pleasant to have people agree with you, too.

Sheila Atchley deserves special recognition. She nudged me two or three times a year for more than 10 years to write a formal statement of continuity theory. She had heard me talk about it in my speeches and workshops many times, and she wanted me to make it more widely available to the field. Her determination to see this happen was perhaps stronger than mine, at least at the beginning. But by 1990, I realized how right she had been. Once the preliminary statement had been written, I had many chances to refine and apply and critique continuity theory in a variety of contexts. This work was an absolute prerequisite for being able to write this book.

I also thank Bob Heinemeyer, Suzanne Kunkel, Sherin Shumavon, Lynn Ritchey, and Debra Stanley, who supervised the various waves of data collection for the OLSAA. Thanks go also to Tina Hartley, Diana Spore, Judith Robinson, and Eileen Root, who as graduate students managed coding, data entry, and data cleaning. Special thanks go to Shahla Mehdizadeh, data manager extraordinaire, who created the file structure and supervised development of an integrated six-wave codebook and the integration of the six survey waves into a single, very large computer file. Thanks also to the many generations of Miami University undergraduate and graduate students who coded, entered, and cleaned data.

I also thank the National Institute of Mental Health and the Ohio Long-Term Care Research Project for funding the OLSAA.

But most of all, I thank the participants in the OLSAA for their patience and willingness to participate throughout such an extended period of time. Without their stories and their ideas, there could be no book.

1 | Continuity Theory

Continuity theory is a theory of continuous adult development, including adaptation to changing situations. In this chapter, I examine how continuity theory evolved, the characteristics of continuity theory as theory, and the specific elements of continuity theory: internal patterns, external patterns, developmental goals, and adaptive capacity. I then consider adult development, especially in later life, and how it differs from aging.

How Did Continuity Theory Arise?

Continuity theory was developed to explain a common research finding: Despite significant changes in health, functioning, and social circumstances, a large proportion of older adults show considerable consistency over time in their patterns of thinking, activity profiles, living arrangements, and social relationships. But the long-term consistency that forms the foundation of continuity theory is not the homeostatic equilibrium predicted by activity theory (Rosow 1967). Instead, continuity is conceived of more flexibly, as strong probabilistic relationships among past, present, and anticipated patterns of thought, behavior, and social arrangements.

Although this book deals with my version of continuity theory (Atchley 1971a, 1989, 1993, 1995, 1997a, 1997b), I was by no means the first to articulate the principle that humans tend to use well-established habits of mind to make sense out of their world and to choose their courses of action (e.g., James 1890). I believe that George Maddox (1968) was the first to apply this principle in gerontology. Based on data from the Duke Longitudinal Study, Maddox observed that over time people tended to maintain their customary lifestyle patterns of activity as they aged. I, too, found that elders tended to maintain patterns of leisure participation across the retirement transition (Atchley 1971a). I also observed that many elders carried their occupational identities with them into retirement. The apparent contradiction between what the conventional academic wisdom of the day said ought to be the relation between identity and behavior (retirement should result in a loss of an occupational identity) and what I and others observed (a carryover of occupational identity into retirement) intrigued and stimulated me to look for underlying social psychological mechanisms. How was it possible that elders were able to maintain a strong and consistent sense of self, high morale, and consistent lifestyle patterns despite presumably major social changes such as retirement, widowhood, or disability?

A high prevalence of continuity in attitudes, beliefs, and values; self-conceptions; social relationships; lifestyles; and environments has been observed by a number of investigators (e.g., Troll 1982; Bengtson et al. 1985; Fiske and Chiriboga 1990; Cohler 1993; Antonucci 1990; Atchley 1997b), so we can be reasonably confident that continuity is a common empirical outcome. However, the prevalence of continuity differs among various dimensions of a person's life. For example, continuity of general personal goals is nearly universal among people as they age; but continuity in feelings of personal effectiveness, of being able to accomplish what one sets out to do, is much less prevalent, especially for those who develop disability as they age. I look at specific examples of continuity over time in later chapters.

Continuity theory takes these empirical findings one step further to attempt to explain why consistency occurs in such a large proportion of cases and over such a large proportion of life domains, sometimes even to the detriment of individual adaptation. Unlike most other theories of adult development that were extensions of child development theories (e.g., Erikson 1963; Levinson 1978), continuity theory was constructed from studies of adaptation in middle-aged and older adults.

That aging brings change is undeniable; so how can we say that continuity is the most prevalent form of adaptation to aging? The key is to conceptualize continuity as the persistence of general patterns rather than as sameness in the details contained within those patterns. Thus, an artist who has spent years drawing and who takes up printmaking is making a change in the details of life as an artist but is showing continuity of commitment to art as an element of self and lifestyle. Likewise, a person who has been religious over an entire lifetime can experience a spiritual deepening that places old values and beliefs in a new context. Religious values and beliefs may remain the same, but the meaning and interpretation that stand behind them evolve. Thus, continuity and change are not mutually exclusive categories that cannot exist simultaneously within an individual self and/or lifestyle. Rather, *continuity and change are themes that usually exist simultaneously in people's lives,* and our challenge is to assess the relative balance between continuity and change at various points in time, over time, and across various life transitions. We should avoid trying to categorize later life as either having continuity or not; both continuity and change are matters of degree, and they coexist. We also need to assess the extent to which people are motivated by a desire for continuity when they make decisions related to goal seeking and adaptation to life changes, including aging-related changes.

To work with continuity theory, we must develop concepts and research methods that differentiate change from continuity. Given that continuity and change usually coexist, the task is to develop sensible decision rules for classifying observed *longitudinal* patterns into patterns dominated by linkage and overall consistency over time and patterns characterized by obvious changes over time.[1]

For example, suppose we are working with the statement "I can do just about anything I set my mind to," and the possible answers to this question are "strongly agree," "agree," "disagree," and "strongly disagree." We asked this question six times over a period of 20 years. People who responded "strongly agree" to all six surveys show absolute stability, which is a form of continuity. But what about people who responded "agree" to three surveys and "strongly agree" to three surveys? I argue that these individuals show continuity because although their level of agreement changed from time to time, they remained in the "agree" conceptual space of the question. By contrast, I would classify respondents who said "strongly agree" to the first four surveys and "disagree" to the last two as showing discontinuity rather than continuity because they shifted from the "agree" conceptual space of the question to the "disagree" conceptual space.

Let us take another example. Suppose we have longitudinal data on the frequency with which respondents participate in 18 types of activity. Those who show the exact same pattern and frequency over time could be classified as showing stability, those who continued to participate in the exact same array of activities but at a slightly lower frequency could be classified as showing continuity, and those who dropped or added a significant number of activities over time could be classified as showing discontinuity.

A third illustration involves classification of scale scores. When measures

---

[1] Cross-sectional data cannot be used to study continuity except by retrospective accounts, which by themselves provide very weak evidence. However, in combination with longitudinal data, retrospective accounts can provide important subjective verification of patterns observed.

consist of aggregated scores on a series of items, we can use data on the mean and standard deviation of the scale to classify longitudinal patterns as showing stability, continuity, or discontinuity. For example, if used with the four-point scale item format mentioned above, the Philadelphia Geriatric Center Morale Scale (Lawton 1975; Morris and Sherwood 1975) consists of 18 items, with a mean score of about 33 and a standard deviation of 4. We can use the standard deviation to assess the degree to which fluctuations in scores for an individual represent stability, continuity, or discontinuity. For instance, an individual who scored 31 on the morale scale for all six waves would obviously fit into the stable category. Another respondent who scored 31, 31, 33, 32, 31, and 33 could be classified as showing continuity because the fluctuations in morale score were well within 1 standard deviation of the individual's initial baseline score. A third respondent who scored 33, 33, 35, 36, 38, and 38 could be classified as showing discontinuity in a positive direction because the pattern of responses showed a steady increase that amounted to more than 1 standard deviation higher than the individual's baseline score.

Conceptually, there are two types of pattern that indicate continuity: absolute stability or lack of change, and overall maintenance of general patterns with minor fluctuations within those patterns. Patterns of discontinuity show dramatic shifts such as ceasing or beginning an activity or shifting from disagreement to agreement with an idea. *Discontinuity focuses on significant departures from past patterns, not minor fluctuations within past patterns.*

Continuity Theory as Theory

As theory, continuity theory is a feedback systems theory (Buckley 1967; Bailey 1990). Feedback systems theories are theories of continuous evolution. The general form of feedback systems theory, as shown in Figure 1.1, presumes that there is an initial pattern that influences behavioral choices or decisions that in turn influence the nature of life experience. Life experience is then used reflexively to evaluate, refine, or revise both the initial pattern and the process of making behavioral choices. This cycle of learning both orientation and behavior from life experience is repeated thousands of times in the course of each year of life. Those who are most open to learning from experience gradually develop over time a highly refined, personalized, and resilient process for anticipating, deciding, and adapting effectively.

Feedback systems theories of adult development assume that people need mental frameworks to organize and interpret their life experiences (Levinson

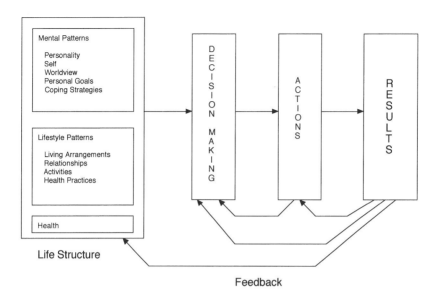

FIGURE 1.1. Continuity as a feedback systems theory.

1990).[2] Individuals have a large array of specific mental frameworks, but continuity theory focuses on global internal frameworks such as the self, personal goals, or belief systems and external patterns such as lifestyles, networks of social relationships, and activity profiles.

Over time, adults develop considerable investment in their conceptions of themselves and the world around them. Individuals are presumed to be dynamic, self-aware entities who use patterns of thought created out of a lifetime of experience to describe, analyze, evaluate, decide, act, pursue goals, and interpret input and feedback. Through their own personal conceptions of how the world is and how it works, their personal strengths and weaknesses, what they are capable of, and what they prefer or dislike, individuals can make effective decisions and thus acquire a sense of personal agency. These conceptions are all present in Buckley's (1967) ground-breaking application of feedback systems theory to social psychology. Continuity theory simply extends these concepts and applies them to development and adaptation in middle and later adulthood.

Continuity theory assumes that the primary goal of adult development is

[2] Levinson was moving toward a systems theory approach in work just before his death. His (1978) initial theory was revised significantly by adding the concept of feedback.

adaptive change, not homeostatic equilibrium. It assumes that adults' patterns of thought about how best to adapt to change continue to develop through learning across the lifespan and that the goal is not to remain the same but to adapt longstanding individual values and preferences to new situations as adults experience life course changes, aging, and social change (Kaufman 1986).

Continuity theory is constructionist. It assumes that in response to their life experiences, people actively develop individualized personal constructs (Kelly 1955), ideas of what is going on in the world and why. Some of our most important personal constructs concern ideas about the self, our relationships with others, and our personal lifestyles. Continuity theory assumes that our personal constructs are *influenced* by the social constructions of reality that we learn from those around us and from the mass media but are not *determined* by them. No matter how strong society's efforts to influence personal constructs, individuals ultimately are free to decide for themselves how to construe their personal reality. An important implication of this aspect of the theory is that *subjective* perceptions of continuity are as theoretically relevant as researchers' perceptions of *objective* continuity.

Continuity theory assumes that patterns of thought and behavior that endure over time are a result of selective investments of time and energy. It posits that people make decisions, based on feedback from experience, about where best to focus their efforts to develop skills and knowledge. People select and develop ideas, relationships, environments, and patterns of activity based on their personal constructs of desired developmental direction and of available opportunity. Individuals invest themselves in the internal and external frameworks of their lives, and these relatively robust frameworks allow individuals to accommodate a considerable amount of evolutionary change without experiencing crisis.

Continuity theory is about adaptation. It presumes that individual choices are made not only to achieve goals but to adapt to constantly changing circumstances, as the individual sees them. Accordingly, continuity theory deals with the development and maintenance of adaptive capacity.

Continuity theory is based on observations of adults in middle age and later life, but it may also apply to the development and maintenance of adaptive capacity in young adulthood as well. Once individuals have developed a strong sense of self, close personal relationships, and a relatively enduring lifestyle, continuity theory can be expected to come into play in explaining their decision-making processes concerning adaptation to life.

Continuity theory is about evolution over the long run, not short-term fluctuations such as changes in mood or transitory forays into new activities. Continuity theory is about the construction and use of enduring patterns designed to enhance life satisfaction and adaptation to change.

If we assume that a primary motive for creating mental frameworks and lifestyle patterns is to allow people to adapt to life circumstances and to pursue life satisfaction, then we would expect individuals to use these highly personalized adaptive structures to make decisions about the future. If effective, decisions based on continuity would reinforce through positive feedback the value of continuity in decision-making strategies. Within most personality types and lifestyle patterns, most people manage to adapt successfully. For example, Williams and Wirths (1965) looked at successful adaptation to aging within several lifestyle types. They found that most elders were able to adapt successfully in most lifestyle types. There was no single lifestyle pattern that was clearly better in terms of leading to successful aging. One interpretation of these findings is that their respondents had selected lifestyles that fit their individual personalities and life goals.

It is also important to acknowledge that continuity theory is not a theory of successful aging, nor is it a deterministic theory that predicts specific outcomes of adaptation. Instead, continuity theory concerns itself with how people attempt to adapt and the mental frameworks they can be expected to use in doing so. Continuity theory does not predict that using a continuity strategy for decision making will lead to successful adaptation; it simply predicts that most people will try continuity as their first adaptive strategy. Continuity theory does not assume that the results of continuity are necessarily positive. The evidence indicates that even those with low self-esteem, abusive relationships, and poor social adaptation resist the idea of abandoning their internal and external frameworks. Apparently, having ground to stand on, even if it predicts a miserable future, is for some people preferable to an unknown future. Similarly, although positive feedback loops may produce positive change, negative feedback loops can produce disorder.

Continuity theory provides a conceptual way of organizing the search for coherence in life stories and of understanding the dynamics that produce basic story lines, but continuity theory has no ideology concerning which stories are "right" or "successful." However, through its diagnostic concepts, continuity theory can help us understand why particular people have developed in the way they have and whether they have adapted well or not.

Nevertheless, continuity strategies seem to be adaptive for a majority of elders, in that these strategies result in maintenance of life satisfaction in most cases, even among those who experience disability (Atchley 1998).

TABLE 1.1. Continuity theory: Assumptions and propositions

Assumptions
— *Continuity* means evolutionary consistency and linkage over time. *Stability* or *equilibrium* is a type of continuity, but evolutionary forms of continuity are more common.
— Continuity over time is commonly observed in the psychological, behavioral, and social patterns of aging individuals.
— Continuity usually coexists with discontinuity.
— Continuity is more evident in general patterns than in the specifics subsumed under general patterns.
— Individual perceptions of reality consist of personal constructs that individuals actively develop by learning from life experience. Culture and socialization influence personal constructs but do not determine them.
— Internal and external patterns of continuity are highly individuated.
— To each individual, what represents continuity is highly subjective.
— Individual patterns of adaptive thought continue to develop throughout life.
— Using continuity strategies to pursue goals or adapt to change does not necessarily lead to successful results, but it does so in a majority of cases.

Propositions
— General patterns of thought, behavior, and relationship are robust and can accommodate considerable change in detailed patterns without triggering a sense of discontinuity.
— Through decision making about self-concept, life course, and lifestyle, and experiencing the consequences, individuals acquire a sense of personal agency.
— Longstanding general patterns of thought, behavior, and relationships result from selective investments of time and attention made by individuals over a period of many years. People are motivated to protect these investments.
— Continuity of general patterns of thought, behavior, and relationships is usually the first strategy people attempt to use to achieve their goals or adapt to changing circumstances.
— Continuity of personal goals provides individuals with an enduring sense of developmental direction.

However, an unyielding desire for continuity can also be maladaptive for individuals who face life changes that cannot be assimilated within what seems to them to be continuity of self and lifestyle. For example, an uncompromising desire for continuity is a major cause of depression connected with entry into nursing homes (Lieberman and Tobin 1983).

Continuity theory is not deterministic. It does not predict specific self or lifestyle content as a result of aging or adaptation. Instead, it tells us where to look to find the internal and external elements people use in adapting to various life circumstances including aging-related changes. Interindividual comparability is in the general form and processes of adaptation, not in the specific outcomes, which are contingent for each individual on his or her specific personal constructs. Similar *types* of social psychological frameworks and processes are presumed to be at work even though they may produce widely varying individual results. The heart of continuity theory is the presumption that people are motivated to continue to use the adaptive strategies they have developed throughout adulthood to diagnose situations, chart future courses, and adapt to change.

Some important basic assumptions and propositions of continuity theory are summarized in Table 1.1.

Elements of Continuity Theory

Using continuity theory requires information on four dimensions of an individual over time: idea patterns, lifestyle, personal goals, and adaptive capacity. Internal continuity can be seen in the maintenance of consistent frameworks of ideas, especially about the self and the phenomenal world. External continuity is expressed in the consistency over time in the social roles, activities, living arrangements, and relationships that make up lifestyle. Personal goals tell us the values the individual wants to actualize as he or she develops. They define an ideal self and an ideal lifestyle that constitute the benchmarks for assessing the results of adaptation. Adaptive capacity can be assessed by looking at the extent to which the person is able to maintain morale in the face of discontinuity.

Internal Patterns

The ideas, mental skills, and information stored in the mind are organized into loose constructs such as self-concept, personal goals, worldview, philosophy of life, moral framework, attitudes, values, beliefs, knowledge, skills, temperament, preferences, and coping strategies. Note that each of these constructs is a general label under which a large number of specific thoughts and feelings can be subsumed. These general frameworks represent different dimensions that, when combined, form a unique whole, distinguishing one person from another. In making life choices and adapting to change, people are motivated to maintain the inner mental constructs that represent a lifetime of selective investment. Ongoing consistency of psychological patterns is viewed by individuals as an important prerequisite for psychological security.

To study continuity of internal mental constructs, we need effective concepts that can be used to develop measures of internal dimensions. Our current models of personality, self, and idea patterns reflect a diversity of viewpoints concerning relevant dimensions. For example, a difficulty in studying continuity in the structure and functioning of the self stems from a lack of agreement on salient dimensions of the self. Each individual has literally hundreds of self-referent ideas. Scholars who study the self thus need to find ways to organize self-referent conceptions into meaningful categories that can be used to aggregate and communicate research results as well as to build theory. Atchley (1982c) organized the self into *self-concept* (objective characteristics of the self), *ideal self* (hoped-for self), *self-values* (personal goals), *self-esteem* (self-liking), and *self-evaluation* (moral self-assessment). Bengtson et al. (1985) added *self-striving* (behavior aimed at creating hoped-for selves and avoiding feared or disvalued selves). Markus and Nurius (1986) introduced the concepts of past, present, and future or *possible selves;* and Rodin and Langer (1977) stressed the importance of *self-agency*, one's perceived capacity to make things happen, as an important support for self-esteem. Wilber (1996) conceived of the development of the self as potentially leading to a *transcendent self.*

Atchley (1982c, 1991) and Markus and Herzog (1991) both conceived of individuals as being active participants in the creation, development, and perpetuation of the structure and dynamics of the self. Markus and Herzog theorized that individuals develop self-schemas that summarize self-referential experience. Examples might include "I can do just about anything I set my mind to" or "I take things hard" or "Having a satisfying job is important to me." These self-schema help the individual interpret and integrate self-referential experience, promote and defend the self, and develop motivation and a sense of developmental direction. Markus and Herzog theorized that self-schema could be influenced by social structural antecedents such as occupation, marital status, race, or gender as well as by life events, social role changes, and changes in health. Markus and Herzog also theorized that psychological well-being and activity patterns could both be seen as results of the structure and dynamics of the self.

External Patterns

Social roles, activities, relationships, living environments, and geographic locations are also organized in a person's mind. As a result of priority setting and selective investment throughout adulthood, by middle age most adults have unique and well-mapped external life situations or lifestyles that differentiate each person from others. Most people attempt to set priorities and make selective investments that will produce the greatest possible satisfaction for them given their constraints. As a result, they see their evolving living arrangements and lifestyle as important sources of social security.

Also, continuity of activities and environments concentrates people's energies in familiar domains where practice can often prevent or minimize the social, psychological, and physical losses that cultural concepts of aging might lead us to expect. Continuity of relationships preserves the network of social support that is important for creating and maintaining solid concepts of self and lifestyle.

Continuity of activities, relationships, and environments has obvious practical advantages, but continuity theory would lead us to expect psychic payoffs as well because external continuity usually involves the actualization of a hoped-for self and avoidance of feared or disvalued selves (Bengtson et al. 1985).

Developmental Goals

Continuity theory assumes that adults have goals for developmental direction: ideals about themselves, their activities, their relationships, and their environments toward which they want to evolve. These personal goals are the focus of self-striving. For example, many older adults place a high priority on spiritual growth and their inner life. Others strive to maintain or improve their family relationships.

Specific developmental goals and even whether people have such goals are influenced by both socialization and location in the social structure — family structure, gender, social class, organizational environment, and so forth. But these goals can also be affected profoundly by life experience. Adults use life experiences to make decisions about selective investments: which aspects of themselves to focus their attention on, which activities to engage in, which careers to pursue, which groups to join, which community to be part of, and so on.

Adaptive Capacity

As they continue to evolve, adults also have increasingly clear ideas about what produces effective decisions and what gives them satisfaction in life, and they intend to fashion and refine an external life situation that complements their internal frameworks and delivers the maximum life satisfaction possible given their circumstances. The ideas that aging adults have about adaptation to life result from a lifetime of learning, adapting, personal evolution, and selective investment, all in interaction or negotiation with their external social and physical environments. When we asked aging adults, "What enables you to cope? What keeps you going?" nearly all easily articulated the resources they use, such as marriage and family relationships, a positive attitude, religiousness, or an attitude of self-reliance and perseverance. It should not be surprising, then, that in adapting to change, adults are motivated to continue to use the internal and external patterns they have spent so much time and energy developing.

Development versus Aging in Later Adulthood

Development can be defined as movement toward evolutionary possibilities (Wilber 1996). Most scholars agree that biological development is completed in young adulthood but also agree that most aging adults retain their capacity for psychological and social growth. For example, psychological development in later adulthood is much more obvious in integrative functions such as wisdom and transcendence rather than in cognitive processes such as mathematical problem solving or psychomotor performance (Baltes 1993). Psychological development also occurs in the process of maintaining adaptive capacity, which may require creativity and ingenuity. Social development in later adulthood can be seen in a shifting of emphasis in relationships from competition to cooperation and from a self-centered orientation to a nurturing attitude toward others (Maehr and Kleiber 1981). Social development is also required if an individual is to assume the caregiving role or the care recipient role successfully. Social development in later adulthood is also influenced by cultural conceptions of what is expected of older adults, which vary widely across various geographic regions and subcultures.

Some psychological and social development in later adulthood is evolutionary growth guided by personal goals; some is evolution stimulated by the need to adapt to aging. *Physical aging* in and of itself is typically a gentle downward slope that can be gradually accommodated to or compensated for with little sense of discontinuity. However, aging increases the probability of multiple chronic health conditions and disability. As we shall see, only in cases of extreme disability does aging result in an experience of more discontinuity than continuity. *Psychological aging* involves modest decrements in cognitive functions, such as learning speed or short-term memory, which typically have little effect on an individual's capacity to function in everyday adult roles. *Social aging* is a paradoxical process that liberates aging adults by freeing them from social role responsibilities but at the same time depreciates their potential contributions. Coping with social aging requires dealing with both increased opportunity and age discrimination, which in turn requires the development and maintenance of a positive self-concept, a workable lifestyle, and a network of social support.

Later life adult development and aging are thus highly interrelated. Although most older adults continue to develop without serious interference from aging, a small but important minority must develop the capacity to deal with significant negative changes that are part of their experience of aging.

Case Examples

I conclude this chapter with several case examples that illustrate three general types of longitudinal pattern: unadulterated continuity, in which physical and mental aging are experienced as a gentle slope, and high morale and lifestyle patterns are maintained; continuity with significant challenge, in which respondents maintain continuity of morale and lifestyle in the face of serious challenges such as widowhood or disability; and discontinuity, in which the psychological patterns and lifestyle integrity present at the beginning of the study have been largely displaced, usually as a result of disability.

I constructed these case studies from three types of longitudinal data: quantitative questionnaire responses, written responses to open-ended questionnaire items, and in-depth interviews with selected respondents.

Unadulterated Continuity: Aging as a Gentle Slope

GWEN AND TED

The Beginning: 1975–1979. When the Ohio Longitudinal Study of Aging and Adaptation (OLSAA) began in 1975 Gwen was 51, and Ted was 57. Both were college graduates. The youngest of their three children was a teenager still living at home. Ted worked as a guidance counselor, a good career choice because he put a high value on helping others. Gwen worked as an administrative troubleshooter in a planning department, which supported her view of herself as someone who could "make things happen." Both were very positive in their attitude toward their work. Gwen thought she would miss her job when the time came to retire, but Ted did not. Gwen also thought that retirement had a negative effect on health, whereas Ted did not. Perhaps as a result, Ted held a completely positive view of their future life in retirement, whereas Gwen was generally positive but with some reservations.

Gwen and Ted were both highly self-confident people, satisfied with their lives, and especially satisfied with the high quality of their marriage. They enjoyed frequent stimulating discussions with one another and often laughed together about life's foibles and experienced good times together. Both described their marriage as practically devoid of negative elements such as sarcasm, anger, criticism, or disagreements.

Although both led busy lives, Gwen's activity level was in the top 10 percent, whereas Ted was exactly average. Part of this difference resulted from the fact that Gwen was much more inclined toward community volunteer work than was Ted, but part also came from the fact that at the beginning of the study Ted was already experiencing some limitations in activity stemming from chronic bronchitis. For example, in 1975 he reported being physically unable to do heavy work around the house. Despite the difference in their activity levels, their activity profiles were remarkably similar. To a great extent, they enjoyed doing the same types of activities at the same frequency.

Ted and Gwen were also quite congruent in terms of their personal goals, especially in their emphasis on close relationships with family and friends and on the premier importance of their relationship with each other. Ted thought that being competent in and satisfied with his work were very important; Gwen thought that these goals were just important. Both were content to be workers in the community, not leaders. Neither placed any importance on hobnobbing with the community elite or on being considered "prominent" in the community.

The Middle: 1979–1981. On the surface, it would seem that a lot had changed for Gwen and Ted between 1979 and 1981. Their youngest child was launched into adulthood, and Ted and Gwen retired when he was 62 and she was 56. Endurance problems connected with bronchitis led Ted to retire earlier than he had planned to in 1975. Health problems also played a role in Gwen's decision to retire early, but she subsequently recovered fully.

Interestingly, neither the empty nest nor retirement seemed to have had a discernible impact on their values, life satisfaction, concepts about themselves, or lifestyle. For both Gwen and Ted, activity levels and patterns remained very consistent before and after these two transitions.

Ted had a very positive attitude toward life in retirement before he actually retired. He envisioned retirement as a time potentially filled with positive experiences — continued involvement, satisfying activity, independence, and freedom. He especially looked forward to the prospect of being able to spend more time with his family, especially his wife. Ted literally saw no negativity at all in the prospect of life in retirement. Gwen's attitude was less positive than was Ted's, but she was still very much in the positive range. Her major concerns were the relationship between retirement and health, which she saw as a great unknown, and her feeling that she might miss her job.

After retirement, Ted's rating of life in retirement became even more positive, and Gwen's rating of it declined slightly, mainly because she saw her life as being slightly less involved and mobile, primarily because of financial constraints on travel. She also saw herself as not being in good health. However, the overall patterns of their attitudes about life in retirement were very consistent across the retirement transition, and both were well above average in their rating of life in retirement. After retirement, Gwen and Ted both downgraded the importance of having a satisfying job. Gwen compensated by raising her priorities on friendships, being independent and self-reliant, and on seeking new experiences. Ted was particularly pleased with his increased opportunity to observe the growth and development of his children and grandchildren.

After retirement, Ted's life revolved around home. He spent much of his time doing yard work, household paperwork, reading, and being with his wife and family. He enjoyed helping his wife with household work and doing things for his children. Gwen's life also revolved around the household and family, but her commitments to volunteer work took her out into the community and created constructive "spaces in our togetherness." Gwen reported that being together more was a good thing that still "took some getting used to." Ted saw the change in totally positive terms, especially doing things together and sharing ideas and experiences. Both reported that retirement had improved an already high-quality marital relationship.

For this couple, the empty nest and retirement had trivial effects on morale, self-concept, values, and lifestyles because they remained in the same house and in the same community. They maintained continuity in their social networks of friends and family, in their community involvements, and in their leisure pursuits. They retained consistent value systems that provided a steady and highly compatible sense of life direction. Retirement enabled them to improve one very important element of their lives — their marriage.

The only dark cloud on the horizon was health related. Although Ted continued the same level of functional capability after retirement as before, he downgraded his self-rated health from good to fair. In addition, Gwen was experiencing minor health problems in 1981. Both Ted and Gwen worried mainly about the future of Ted's worsening chronic bronchitis and its potential effect on their life together.

Later: 1991–1995. By 1995, Ted's steadily worsening bronchitis had severely limited what he was physically able to do. He reported that mundane things such as carrying groceries to the car or from the car to the house became something he had to think about and take more slowly. He could no longer perform activities that took sustained physical effort, such as washing the car, cleaning out the garage, or weeding the garden. Climbing stairs became very time consuming. Given the limitations he faced, Ted's activity level and profile changed remarkably little. Like most retirees, he ceased being involved in occupational organizations, and he reduced his political activities. However, he increased his involvement in community service by joining Gwen in some of her volunteer efforts. For example, he drove the car while she delivered Meals on Wheels to elders in the community. By 1995, Ted spent much more time resting than in 1991. Gwen had returned to good health by 1991, and she remained so through 1995.

Despite the changes in Ted's health, neither he nor Gwen reported any change in their morale, self-confidence, positive view of life in retirement, or marital satisfaction. Ted compensated for activities he could do less frequently by increasing his focus on the growth and development of young people and enjoying "the miracles of nature" and engaging in stimulating conversation with his large network of family and friends. He seems to have focused less on doing and more on relating. Indeed, Ted's primary means of coping was to "quietly give love" to those around him, primarily in the form of attention and care. Thus, his longstanding priority on relationships sustained him very well in the face of physical changes.

Although Ted experienced major changes in what he was physically able to do, he was not disabled in terms of either ordinary adult functioning or Activities of Daily Living (ADL).[3] Gwen coped with these changes through social support from her family and her religious faith. In our most recent survey, Ted and Gwen still had marital satisfaction scale scores well above average, even in a panel in which most couples were very happily married.

Continuity played a very critical role in preserving positive attitudes, strong interpersonal relationships, and satisfying lifestyles for this couple. Gwen and Ted both felt that they knew themselves well enough to make sound decisions about what to do and not do, that their choices produced the results they expected and led to their strengths and avoided their weaknesses, and that past solutions were a sound guide for current decision making. In short, they perceived the inner and outer continuity that characterized their lives as being the intentional results of their past decisions and actions.

From the beginning of our study, Gwen and Ted were active, self-confident, interested people with a strong marriage and plenty of friends and family with whom to exchange social support. The viewpoints and lifestyles that they had created even before our study began allowed them to cope easily with the empty nest and retirement and to experience aging as a gentle slope despite Ted's deteriorating health. Even with his health-imposed activity limitations, Ted's activity level remained about average for the panel in 1995, mainly because he was broadly engaged to begin with and could offset losses with increases in other activity areas. Ted and Gwen illustrate very clearly the positive results that can come from constructing a viable approach to living life and sticking with it.

[3] Activities of Daily Living such as bathing, dressing, eating, ambulating, using the toilet, and getting into and out of a bed or chair are often used to measure the extent of disability and need for long-term care in the older population.

DALE

The Beginning: 1975–1979. At the beginning of our study, Dale was 57. His work involved calling on schools within a 60-mile radius to sell kitchen equipment and to arrange to have kitchen equipment refurbished. He enjoyed his work. His wife worked as a secretary at the local university. They had three adult children, all of whom lived within a 30-minute drive of their small but comfortable home.

Dale's life revolved around his employment, work around the house, and activities with his wife. He and his wife made trips in their recreational vehicle almost every weekend during good weather, and they visited many different parts of the surrounding country. They also enjoyed bowling, golfing, and fishing. Dale spent the remainder of his free time visiting with family and watching television.

He was extremely satisfied with the quality of his marriage. He reported that he and his wife worked together quite frequently, particularly gardening and accomplishing the logistics for their trips. They also engaged in frequent discussions, laughed often, and had a good time together. Dale and his wife had occasional disagreements, but they were almost never sarcastic, critical, or standoffish with one another.

Dale was in good health throughout the study, and only in 1995, at age 77, did he report that his endurance was no longer up to full-time employment. His score was very high on all preventive health measures.

He had very high self-confidence, high morale, and a very positive attitude toward the prospects of retirement.

Later: 1981–1995. Dale retired in 1980, but he continued to work part-time for the same company through 1991, mainly during the company's busiest periods. He felt that retirement had improved an already strong marriage, and he believed that the increased time he and his wife spent together resulted in greater intimacy.

His activities remained remarkably consistent over the entire 20-year study period. He offset slight reductions in gardening, television watching, participatory sports, and time spent with family and friends by increases in travel, attending sporting events, and reading. His basic array of activities remained unchanged, including his total lack of involvement in hobbies or in local organizations, including church.

Dale's health continued to be good. He developed a heart condition in 1992, had a bypass operation, and was fully recovered by 1995. At 77, he was in good health and able to perform all of the functional activities on our scale except working at a full-time job.

His attitude toward life in retirement, which was above average in 1975, was among the most positive in the study by 1995. Retirement had very definitely lived up to his expectations. He reported only very minor fluctuations in morale and self-confidence throughout the study, and both remained above average.

Dale's main goals in life were modest: to remain in good health, to have a close relationship with his wife, to remain in their home, and to enjoy their activities together. When asked how he coped with life's ups and downs, he said, "with a positive attitude and a wonderful wife." His strategy of focusing his life around his marriage very definitely worked for Dale. His attention to preventive health practices also was effective. He scored very high on our scale of predisposition toward continuity, and his responses indicated that he perceived his life as having a high degree of continuity, which matched our longitudinal research data. He saw his continuity of attitudes, values, relationships, and activities as being the result of his own planning and conscious decisions. Dale is an example of someone who wanted continuity very much and whose good health, intact marriage, and modest but adequate retirement income provided every opportunity to realize this goal. Thus far, Dale has experienced aging as a very gentle slope with no serious challenges to his preferred ways of thinking, relating, and living.

Substantial Change with Positive Outcome

EDNA

The Beginning: 1975–1977. Edna was age 72 when the study began in 1975. She had graduated from college in 1924 and in 1950 earned her Masters degree in education. She had been retired for two years from a very satisfying career as a home economics teacher. She had enjoyed teaching, and she felt that she had made a very positive contribution to her students, many of whom came from economically and socially deprived backgrounds.

Edna was widowed in 1948 and did not remarry. Her two sons were ages 10 and 15 when their father died, and she was proud that they had "turned out very well." Throughout the study, she continued to live alone in a small, cozy house located in a busy neighborhood and near the public library and shopping areas.

Edna was a highly independent, self-confident woman who took a great deal of satisfaction from her life experiences. She was very active, strove to improve herself, and had a very positive attitude toward her life in retirement. Even though she lived alone, she had more than 15 friends who lived in her community and with whom she maintained frequent contact. She loved attending social gatherings, and her cooking skills meant that she could be counted on to contribute to community bake sales, of which there were many. She was active in her political party at the county level, and she frequently attended meetings of the retired teachers association. She also traveled frequently to spend time with her family — each of her sons and their families lived two to three hours away. She felt it was easier for her to drive to visit them because "there is only one of me to worry about; you know, schedules and all that."

Edna was emphatic in her feelings that if people had bad experiences in retirement "it's their own fault." She believed that planning for retirement and the contingencies of old age was the key to a satisfying life. She put these opinions into practice. She made careful financial plans for retirement and had a comfortable but modest income. She also was a strong believer in preventive health practices. The only preventive health practice on our scale that she did not observe faithfully was watching her weight, which had never been a problem for her. She was also a strong believer in approaching life with a positive attitude.

Edna believed that she had gotten got a good start in life, especially from the faith and teachings of her grandmother. Through these early experiences she developed a habit of appreciating and being grateful for her life. When we first interviewed Edna, the familiar expression "I am the captain of my fate and the master of my soul" described our overall impressions of her. Over the next 20 years, she maintained this viewpoint to good advantage.

The Middle: 1981. By 1981, arthritis had begun to limit Edna's mobility. She found climbing stairs arduous, which made it more difficult for her to go out of her home. But she continued to make the effort and was still very active in the community. Her overall activity level remained unchanged. However, her physical difficulties took their toll on her self-confidence, especially on her assessment of her capacity to pursue her goals. Her self-confidence dropped from very high to average for the women in the panel. Nevertheless, her morale remained very high, and her attitude toward her life in retirement was still very positive. She maintained a very high degree of consistency over time in her attitudes, values, activities, and relationships.

Her major goals at this stage were "to continue to be alert and helpful, to enjoy the privileges of friendship, to protect my health, and to appreciate my family ties." Her outgoing, appreciative attitude was an important factor in her ability to maintain her contacts with friends and participation in the community despite her physical mobility problems.

Later: 1991–1995. By 1991, Edna's physical mobility problems had worsened considerably, but at age 88 she still maintained her very positive outlook on life. She fell in 1990 and broke a hip, had hip replacement surgery, and went through a consequent period of slightly reduced activity in 1991. The fall that broke her hip also produced nerve damage in one leg that caused a loss of coordination that could not be recovered. She had to use a walker and canes to get around the house, so going out for groceries, to the doctor, to community gatherings, and so on became even more difficult. But by 1995, at age 92, with help she was almost as active as she had been 20 years earlier.

She adapted her lifestyle to her more homebound state by doing less gardening and cutting back her participation in politics and in community organizations. However, she increased participation in senior center activities, spent more time with her collection of family photographs and memorabilia, and watched more television—mainly educational programs focused on the arts, nature, or public affairs.

When Edna could not perform as much community service as she had before, she shifted her focus to self-improvement. She believed that television had become an important and new vehicle for continuing to exercise her mind and improve herself. In her usual strong-willed fashion, she said, "I don't use TV to just pass time. I use it to keep mentally sharp."

Edna hired a person to help her with housework while she was recovering from her fall and surgery. "She wasn't a very good housekeeper, but I found that she was good company and quite willing to help me get around. I can't drive any more, so she helps me to my car and walks with me through [the grocery]. I use the shopping cart as a sort of walker, but I still like having her there in case I can't reach something." She showed excellent dexterity in using a special three-wheeled walker with handbrakes.

Adapting to her changing mobility was a major goal for Edna, and she accomplished this goal with her usual positive approach, planning, and creativity. In 1995, Edna still had very high morale, a realistic appraisal of her personal agency, and a very active and satisfying life. She enjoyed her memories from "a stimulating and satisfying career," and she appreciated having so many "younger" friends (most of whom were over 60). Her sons were 57 and 62, and she followed the development of her grandchildren and great-grandchildren with much interest. Edna's religious faith was a major resource for coping. She was never a frequent churchgoer, but she had a deep and abiding trust in God that she had learned from her grandmother and that had nurtured her throughout her life. She participated very frequently in reciprocal social support with her many friends, and she believed in keeping busy; to do so in her housebound state, she volunteered to be an interview subject for college students, thus initiating a series of new experiences and relationships delivered to her door.

At 92, Edna was still very much in charge of her life and making the most of it. She retained her strong sense of direction, although she understood that there were events beyond her control to which she would have to adapt. But she knew herself and what worked for her. She was not afraid of death, she enjoyed her inner life more than when she was 50, and she felt a greater connection to the universe. Even though she had to adapt to substantial physical disability, she did so successfully. Looking back, she saw her life as having a very high degree of continuity of basic values, interpersonal relationships, and lifestyle. This assessment was strongly confirmed in our longitudinal data.

For Edna, continuity of activities and lifestyles was not always possible, but she used great planning, intelligence, and creativity to cope with significant changes and to maintain the basic patterns of thinking and acting that had been her hallmark all along. Continuity is not merely inertia but often the result of highly motivated and intentional action. Edna wanted continuity, and she proceeded to create the conditions necessary to produce it.

GILES

The Beginning: 1975–1977. In 1975, Giles was age 51 and living with his wife of 25 years. They had three grown children who lived in distant parts of the country. Giles held a graduate degree in art and worked as a painter and as an art teacher. He did not find his teaching situation satisfying, and he looked forward to retiring from it. His wife was an administrator at a local university. Giles was satisfied with his marriage, especially the high degree of intimacy he and his wife enjoyed. He was a stoic respondent who rarely checked the most positive end of any continuum; he always thought there was room for improvement.

Giles's activity level was below average because he was very selective in what he did. He was deeply engaged in maintaining very close relationships with his wife and children, painting, listening to music, keeping up on politics, enjoying nature, reading, and exercising. Apart from politics, he participated only to a very modest extent in local organizations. He seldom attended church functions. He was only occasionally interested in hobbies or crafts. Although Giles did not find his job satisfying, his strong work ethic meant that he invested a great amount of time in his teaching, and he took a great interest in his students.

Giles's morale and self-confidence fluctuated from time to time, depending on the situation in his family and on his job. In 1975 his morale and self-confidence were above average, but by 1977 his sister had died unexpectedly, his responsibility for the care of his mother had increased, and he had not secured a job promotion he had sought. These circumstances created a situation in which his morale and self-confidence were lowered significantly.

Giles was very positive about his prospective life in retirement. He looked forward to no longer having to be involved in an undesirable work situation. He was also "fed up with politics" and wanted to withdraw gradually from what had been a significant involvement. He anticipated an active, involved, and meaningful retirement in which he would be free to pursue his own agenda. He planned to retire several years earlier than did his wife.

Giles was in good health, and he had no functional impairments or activity limitations. However, he scored low on preventive health measures such as watching his diet and weight, moderate alcohol consumption, and getting a regular physical.

His goals centered on his family. He was an unselfish husband and father, and he often put his family ahead of himself. He kept himself well informed on politics and enjoyed the company of an informal group of men who met regularly for breakfast. He strove to make sure the family would have a comfortable income, and he believed that being able to accept himself was very important. He did not consider religion or community prominence important at all.

The Middle: 1979–1981. Giles's activity level increased considerably during this period. He spent much more time on his painting, he and his wife traveled frequently and began to assemble a collection of antiques and art from many countries, and he began to write a book on funding for the arts. He continued to read widely to keep up on politics. He reported fewer in-person contacts with his children, but he and his wife were frequently in touch with each of them by telephone.

By 1981, his job situation had become even worse, and he saw his job career as a disappointing one in which he had not been able to live up to his own expectations. He took early retirement in 1984 at age 60, five years earlier than he had planned in 1979. He retired six years earlier than did his wife, who continued to work full time until 1990. He envisioned retirement as a welcome permission to become less involved not only in his job but also in various community activities. His attitude toward retirement remained very positive, but he began to have concerns about his health, although he continued to rate his health as good and had no functional impairments or chronic diseases. He also was concerned about finances in retirement because of the high inflation that characterized the 1979–81 period.

His concerns about health in retirement were probably related to the health of his mother, for whom he continued to be a primary caregiver, doing household chores, providing transportation, and visiting. Her health deteriorated during this period, and his caregiving responsibilities increased accordingly. He also had to provide financial support to his mother, which heightened his awareness of the expense of being frail and increased his concerns about his own retirement income.

Giles's morale remained average and his self-confidence below average during this period. His major goals were to serve his family, keep well informed, protect the family income, be reliable, and accept himself as he was.

Later: 1991–1995. By 1991, Giles's life had changed considerably. He had retired in 1984 and experienced several very enjoyable years of freedom in retirement. Although his wife continued to work, he kept himself occupied with his painting and his informal contacts with his many friends. He also continued to play tennis and golf. As he had planned, he cut back sharply on his participation in local politics. He most definitely did not miss his job. His mother had died, freeing him from his caregiving responsibilities. He and his wife were able to travel more often, and they continued to add to their art collection.

However, in 1990 he was diagnosed as having a particularly virulent form of cancer, and he was told that he had only months to live. He endured several surgeries, radiation treatments, and chemotherapy over a period of nearly a year. But the result was successful. By 1992 his cancer was in remission, and as of 1995 he had had no recurrence.

His understandable preoccupation with his health caused a noticeable reduction in his activity level, but he gave up none of his customary activities entirely. The surgeries excised considerable muscle tissue, which made it difficult for him to paint or to play golf or tennis as much as he had before, but he continued to exercise, gather strength, and compensate for the physical changes. Gradually he was able to maintain these activities, albeit at a lower level than before. He also cut back on gardening, handiwork, collecting, attending social gatherings, and even watching television.

Interestingly, his self-confidence increased at this time, perhaps because he was taking an active stance in relation to his recovery from cancer. Having "beaten cancer," his morale had also increased. His relationship with his wife became even closer, probably related to the increased care, social support, and attention she had provided during his illness. He viewed his marriage as extremely satisfying. Despite his illness, his psychological well-being in 1991 was at a high point.

However, in 1993, Giles's wife was diagnosed with ovarian cancer, which had spread to her lymph system. Despite surgery and a series of other treatments, her health declined rapidly, and Giles spent much of 1993 and 1994 caring for her at home. Although this situation was certainly not what they had planned for their retirement, Giles saw himself as having to be "strong as a rock" to care for his wife, and he was able to live up to his own expectations. Nevertheless, he was plagued by anxiety because his life revolved around his wife, and she was clearly terminal. She died in the late summer of 1994.

Outwardly, Giles's life remained much the same after his wife's death. He continued to travel frequently, particularly to visit his children, other relatives, and long-time friends. He increased the frequency of his telephone contacts with his children significantly. He continued to be part of an informal breakfast group that discussed various goings-on in the community, he continued to exercise, he spent more time reading and much more time watching sports and news on television. His other activities remained at their previous levels.

But inwardly, Giles was in shambles. He had trouble sleeping. He had difficulty sitting still for any length of time. He felt that his life in retirement, which had been so positive, was now bad, inactive, and sad. He felt sick, even though his physical health was good. He was lonely much of the time, and even though he kept busy and tried to maintain a positive attitude, he was clearly still grieving and was not satisfied with his life. Despite these profound experiences, his morale dropped only slightly, and his new-found self-confidence was a resource he could use to cope. As he said, "I try to preserve my own health by exercising and leading a healthy life, and I focus on keeping busy and on being helpful to my children."

Giles had experienced significant discontinuities during the study period, especially related to caregiving for his mother, his own life-threatening illness, and his wife's terminal illness and death. Yet through all of this, he had maintained considerable continuity in his activities, relationships with family and friends, and approach to life. He also continued to live in the same home throughout the study. And despite the obvious downturn in some aspects of psychological well-being connected with the grieving process, he continued to adopt his usual stoic stance toward whatever life brought. He was committed to getting through it.

In an open-ended interviewed in 1997, Giles was obviously still grieving for his wife. He continued to live alone, keep busy, travel a lot, and focus his attention on the needs of his children. He was sleeping better but was still lonely much of the time. We got a clear impression that he was coming to terms with his new life. He was using a continuity strategy to cope. He said that he used his knowledge of himself, strategies that had worked for him in the past, time-tested satisfying activities, and a clear life philosophy to maintain his continuity of lifestyle, morale, and self-confidence. He was sure that he would eventually adapt to life as a widower.

Unwanted Discontinuity with Negative Outcomes

MIKE AND ELAINE

The Beginning: 1975–1981. When our study began, Mike was 55 and employed as a professor at the local university. Elaine was 53 and director of a local social service agency. They had three children, all of whom had been launched into adulthood. Both enjoyed their jobs very much, and they focused their lifestyle around employment. They were among the few OLSAA respondents who spontaneously listed "work" as one of their most frequent activities — most people listed activities other than employment.

Over the 1975–81 period, both members of this couple showed a high degree of consistency in activities, psychological well-being, and goals. When he was not teaching, Mike did woodworking, watched television, and read. Elaine's most important activities were playing music, gardening, and participating in a variety of political, service, and professional organizations in the community. Both reported that they frequently spent time with friends and family, and they traveled often.

Both enjoyed positive psychological well-being. Elaine was about average for the panel on self-confidence, morale, and attitude toward life in retirement, which is to say that she was generally positive. Mike, on the other hand, had very high self-confidence, average morale, and a higher than average positive view of the prospects of life in retirement.

Mike's goals revolved around self-acceptance and being with family. Elaine was concerned with maintaining good health, self-improvement, and helping others, especially her family.

At the beginning of the study, Mike and Elaine were not sure if they would ever retire, although both expected that the quality of their life in retirement would be quite positive. Elaine felt that being together more would enhance the quality of their relationship.

From 1975 to 1981, both Mike and Elaine continued their customary lifestyles, and they each experienced aging as a gentle downward slope that required little conscious adaptation. Mike experienced some minor limitations in his activities because of asthma, but neither his overall activity level nor his psychological well-being was affected.

Later: 1991–1995. In 1987, Mike and Elaine retired and moved from Ohio to a distant Sunbelt state. Their choice of destination was determined in part by the fact that one of their sons and his family lived in that area. Both had expected their retirement to be active, involved, and healthy and to involve greater companionship.

However, Elaine bought a partnership interest in a local retail franchise, and in 1991 her activities were centered on the needs of this business. She was very busy working in the store, attending work-related events, and doing business-related paperwork. She reported a significant reduction in seven activities she had enjoyed before the move, especially involvement in community organizations.

Meanwhile, Mike's asthma continued to restrict his activities mildly, and the move from their community of long residence resulted in a significant drop in his activity level, from average in 1981 to significantly below average in 1991. His major activities were cooking and "fixing things" around the house. He missed woodworking, gardening, travel, and frequent visits with family and friends. Elaine said, "Since I continue to work and meet new people, I feel a certain guilt and frustration because he is home alone in a strange community and doesn't seem to have the initiative to get out and make a new life for himself." At this stage, Mike still rated his marriage as extremely satisfying. Elaine rated her marriage as satisfying but not extremely so.

By 1995, Elaine had given up her involvement in the business, in part because she needed to provide caregiving to her husband. She said, "We have too much togetherness sometimes. His physical limitations reduce our ability to do much outside the home. We can't travel because of his physical limitations, and I feel that I should stay and take care of him, so I can't travel by myself." However, Mike did not have significant functional impairments. He could not do heavy work around the house or maintain a full-time job or walk a half-mile, but he could walk up and down stairs, go out into the community, and do ordinary housework. Mike's asthma was troublesome but not severe, and he had no other disabling health conditions, so it was unclear what care he required other than companionship.

Elaine felt that things were much worse than she had expected; she wished they still lived in Ohio near their friends, she felt lonely a lot of the time, she was not satisfied with how she spent her free time, and she was unhappy with her life in general. Mike's unwillingness to leave the house had restricted her to the household, which in turn caused her to reduce even further nine activities in which she had been involved frequently in 1981. Not surprisingly, compared with 1981, her self-confidence and morale had both dropped to below average, and her view of life in retirement had changed from very positive to much less so, especially in terms of feeling that her life in retirement was uninvolved, helpless, and meaningless.

Mike's activity level had declined even further by 1995; his major activities consisted of watching television, feeding the birds, and helping his wife. He continued to perform very few of the activities that made up his lifestyle in 1981. His morale and self-confidence dropped to significantly below average, and the very positive view of retirement he had held earlier was challenged by new perceptions of sickness, uninvolvement, and idleness.

Both Mike and Elaine seem to have significantly underestimated how much they would miss the social support from the friends they left behind in Ohio. Even though they had family nearby, Mike's increasingly homebound lifestyle caused a significant drop in frequency of interaction with them.

Elaine coped with her situation by relying on her feeling of connection with God and spiritual sources of inspiration, such as books and tapes. She also used social support from family to help her cope. Despite her frustrations with caregiving and what she saw as her husband's lack of initiative, Elaine also continued to see their relationship as an important coping resource. Mike, on the other hand, cited "sense of humor" as his only coping resource. Perhaps because Elaine was there to provide the support he needed, he was more satisfied than she was with their marriage and with their life in general.

Mike and Elaine are a clear case of discontinuity far outweighing continuity. Their life before retirement was active and satisfying, and both of them were self-confident and satisfied with their life together. But a combination of moving to a new community, Elaine's involvement in a new business, and Mike's increasing dependence combined to alter the structure and rhythm of their lives completely. Before, they were independent and active, and Elaine was very involved in the community. After, Mike was increasingly dependent, and Elaine was constrained more and more to life within their home, which was especially unsatisfying to her. Neither of them preferred this new life, as indicated by their significant declines in morale and self-confidence, but they felt helpless to do anything about it. Interestingly, Mike and Elaine both scored low on the disposition toward continuity scale, and the low priority they placed on continuity does not seem to have served them well.

DOLORES

The Beginning: 1975–1977. In 1975, Dolores was 71. She was married and living with her husband in a large comfortable home near the campus of the college where he had been employed. He had retired three years earlier. Despite having graduated from college and having completed a graduate degree, Dolores was of the generation of women whose "career" consisted of being a full-time homemaker and mother. She was employed for only a few years in young adulthood; after her first son was born in the 1930s, she never again held a paying job. Each of her two sons lived in very distant states.

Dolores was very sensitive about what she considered to be the depreciated status of full-time homemakers, and she was not sure how our questions about retirement applied to her. Because her husband continued to do consulting work and she retained her identity as a homemaker, she wondered how the concept of retirement applied to them. Nevertheless, it was clear that they were very positive about the freedom and flexibility that retirement income and self-employment offered. Even in retirement, their household income was among the highest in the study. She also appreciated the additional time together that her husband's retirement had allowed. Her concept of the good life very definitely revolved around being part of a couple, and she was extremely satisfied with the quality of her marriage.

Dolores was very active, well above average for all of the women in the panel. She and her husband were "snowbirds," who spent the winter months in Florida, where she especially enjoyed the warmth of the sun, which helped her arthritis. She was involved in a wide variety of informal activities, including socializing with friends and social gatherings, but she did not participate in community organizations often. From our list of 16 specific personal goals, she felt that being well read and informed was the only one that was very important to her. Being useful, primarily to her family but also to a lesser extent to her neighborhood and community, was a major organizing principle in her life. Although she had many acquaintances, she felt that forming close, long-lasting friendships was unimportant, which probably made the snowbird lifestyle more attractive.

Dolores had a modestly positive attitude toward life in retirement; she was concerned about her health and had a feeling of not being involved. Indeed, she already had minor health problems, particularly arthritis in her spine, which limited her ability to stoop or climb many stairs and to do heavy work around the house. She rated her health as only fair.

Despite these difficulties, she was very self-confident, and her morale was high. But Dolores was very vocal about the difficulties of finding adequate domestic help. "On some of our travels, we meet people who call themselves 'cruisers' who spend months on long cruises because all of their needs — cooking, cleanup, grocery shopping, entertainment, housekeeping, transportation, etc. are taken care of. They cannot get this at home 'for love nor money.' Most of them have sold their big houses and live in condominiums where they need only to lock the door when they want to go away for any length of time. Living gracefully in a servantless home is a thing of the past."

The Middle: 1979–1981. During this period, Dolores remained in the same home and remained extremely satisfied with her married life in retirement. Her life focus was on being independent and retaining her "faculties" — eyesight, memory, hearing. She spent a great deal of time corresponding with her family in order to maintain close ties with them.

Her functional capability continued to decline gradually. By 1979, she could no longer walk a half-mile, and she reported that her spinal arthritis had curtailed her mobility further. However, Dolores's activities dropped only slightly, mostly gardening, attending sporting events, and handiwork. She and her husband continued wintering in Florida, and they made several trips abroad. She was still enjoying a retirement lifestyle focused on activities that she and her husband did together. She remarked that since retirement, her husband participated much more with her in gardening and helped her with shopping. She also enjoyed the intimacy she felt when they were spending time together.

Dolores's morale continued at baseline level, which was high. However, her self-confidence dropped significantly, mainly because of the effects of increased mobility limitations on her concept of personal agency. She accepted that there were limits on what she could accomplish physically. She also perceived that her life involved a slight degree of chronic sickness.

Later: 1991–1995. Dolores was 87 in 1991, and her life had changed considerably since 1981. After her husband's death in 1988, she moved from her home of many years to a condominium in the same town. Her health continued to deteriorate, and by 1995 she was essentially homebound. She went from being impaired but still independent to being dependent on paid caregivers and household workers.

In 1991, she could get around the house using crutches or a walker, and she could still drive. She had broken her hip in a fall and had had hip replacement surgery, which was not altogether successful. Her sciatic nerve was damaged, and she reported being in constant pain. She also had to have surgery for carpal tunnel syndrome in her right wrist, which "made it difficult to use a crutch or walker and ruined my handwriting." Being right-handed, she also found it more difficult to use handrailings. She went out much less "because most buildings are inaccessible to me. Even if I can get to [the music hall], the restrooms often require being able to go up and down stairs." In addition, she was bothered by failing eyesight and hearing.

Dolores found many other disadvantages to her increased level of disability. She said that "the worst problem about being handicapped is getting groceries." The two stores that delivered charged fees that to her seemed outrageous. In addition, the post office would not deliver mail to her door, and she had to pay extra to have her newspaper placed inside her storm door. When she could get out, she was frustrated. The handicapped parking spaces were often located in such a way that she had to cross an intersection, and the traffic lights did not allow sufficient time for her to do so. She did appreciate the fact that her new condominium was completely accessible — all one floor, with no stairs.

Dolores cut back significantly on travel because of the discomfort involved in sitting for too long. She did remark that "for a handicapped person, the travel people provide a level of help that I cannot regularly get at home. They send someone to pick me up, get me on the plane, meet me, and get me home." She had hired three helpers to do housework, prepare some of her meals, help her bathe, and sometimes help her in and out of bed. She also employed people to manage her money and do her gardening. She remained very much in charge of her situation, frustrating as it was to her.

Dolores still tried to remain active, but her focus now was on reading, watching television, cooking, and planning activities for the hired gardener. Instead of writing, she maintained contacts with family by telephone. She missed her husband a great deal. She also missed their active lifestyle — the winters in Florida and travel to faraway places. She missed being able to get out into the community even to the limited extent she had enjoyed in 1981. Dolores's activity loss was profound. In 1975, she had been involved at least to some extent in all 18 activity areas covered in our survey. By 1991, she had completely ceased seven activities and did another five only rarely. Her overall activity level dropped from above average to one of the lowest in the panel.

Given her losses — her husband's death, her increased disability, and the loss of valued activities — it is no surprise at all that Dolores experienced a further significant drop in self-confidence and a significant drop in morale.

By 1995, at age 91, Dolores could no longer walk. Even with assistance, she required a brace on her left leg. She rated her health as poor because in addition to her mobility and pain problems, she had developed recurrent angina, a painful heart condition. She said, "The angina limits my ability to reach high above my head and picking up anything on the floor."

Her activity level had dropped even further. She occupied herself by corresponding and talking on the telephone with friends and family, reading, watching television, and bird watching ("My helpers keep the bird feeders filled"). She was unsatisfied with the way she was spending her time but felt she had little choice. Her life was shadowed by images of her life "when I was 20 years younger, in good health, and had my dear husband with me, both of us healthy and able to travel and enjoy life and visit our children."

Dolores's self-confidence and morale remained very low, for understandable reasons — widowhood, disability, activity limitations, chronic pain. In addition, she felt that her life in retirement, which had been so positive earlier, had become filled with a sense of sickness, disability, helplessness, emptiness, and meaninglessness. She frequently felt lonely and was very unsatisfied with her life.

Nevertheless, she was grateful for the few friends who came to visit. She had outlived most of her friends. She also appreciated the work that her three paid helpers provided. She was very grateful for having the economic means to pay the number of people she required to support her being able to stay in her independent household. She was also satisfied with the quality of help she was getting. She felt that she continued to contribute to the community by providing financial support to the charity work of community organizations.

Dolores coped with her situation mainly by using her material resources to maintain some semblance of control and continuity within her household. As the external structure of her life disintegrated, she had fragile self-confidence or social support upon which to draw. She had no deeply held faith, she found no enjoyment in an inner life, she felt no connection with the universe, so internal religious coping was not an option for her.

Dolores is a clear case of discontinuity. Her physical capability declined gradually for many years and then declined precipitously. Her husband's death destroyed the dyadic household structure around which her life had revolved successfully for more than 60 years. Her increased disability isolated her more and more from interaction outside her household. Her sense of physical, mental, and social well-being in 1995 was extremely negative, whereas in 1975 even her health had been at least positive, and she enjoyed high morale, self-confidence, and a large array of satisfying activities done frequently. She herself confirmed that compared with 1985, her basic lifestyle, her friends, and even her basic values had changed significantly.

Unwanted Discontinuity with Positive Outcomes

JANE

The Beginning: 1975–1981. In 1975, Jane was 52 and at the top of her field as a full professor and chair of her department at a local university. She had never married, and she had no children. She maintained close ties with her family, and she had many close friends in the community.

Jane's life revolved around service to others. She put a high priority on her teaching and administrative work at the university, and she also took an active role in regional and national professional organizations in her field. She was active in several community organizations, especially her church, was an avid gardener, and enjoyed many opportunities to travel. She had an active social life, attending many social gatherings and visiting with friends very frequently. During this period, when she was 52 to 58, her overall activity level remained among the highest in the panel.

Jane was a highly self-confident woman with very high morale and an extremely positive attitude toward her prospective life in retirement. There was literally no area of life in retirement that she did not see in completely positive terms, but she felt exactly the same way about her current life. Her worldview was rooted in a spiritual life of disciplined inner inquiry and enthusiastic participation in her church.

She found value in all of the personal goals in our list of 16. Her own list stressed "being a useful member of society, being both respected and loved, having a comfortable life, being an active member of the community, and being dependable."

She followed all of the prevention steps to ensure good health, and she rated her health as very good throughout this period. She reported that she had taken no medications in more than 20 years.

In 1988, Jane retired at age 65. However, in keeping with her past record, she continued to serve the university, using her many contacts with former students to encourage increased alumni contributions. She served the community by being elected to the city council, where she served with her usual enthusiasm. Before 1990, Jane seemed destined to experience aging as a process of very gentle change characterized by continued good health, satisfying activity, and distinguished service to the community.

The Middle: Catastrophe. In 1992, Jane began to experience severe pain in her hip. After a lengthy series of tests, doctors diagnosed her as suffering from bone cancer that had spread throughout her body. Her oncologist did not expect her to live another six months. She underwent radiation and chemotherapy and endured excruciating pain. She moved from her comfortable home to a skilled nursing facility in a nearby town where, as a person medically defined as dying, she was given eligibility for Medicare hospice services.

Jane maintained her positive outlook, and she prevailed against seemingly insurmountable odds. Although she was left unable to walk by the aggressive cancer therapy, by 1994 she was cancer free. In late 1994, she lapsed into a coma. Again she was not expected to live, but she recovered. In 1995, she continued to participate in our survey.

Later: The Aftermath: 1995–1997. Although Jane had experienced drastic negative changes in her physical health and appearance, functional capability, living arrangements, social relationships, and pattern of activities, her morale and self-confidence remained very high in 1995. However, she was not a Pollyanna. Her rating of her life in retirement realistically acknowledged her sickness and her dependence. She understood fully that she had lost many valued activities, and she wished she could still perform them. But inside that disabled body, her inner faith and positive outlook remained strong. She said, "I get up in the morning ready to make the most of everything the day offers. I take part in all the activities to keep my mind stimulated. Given my previous life, I never though I'd be playing Bingo, but I always try to find something good in my experiences here [in the retirement community where she still lives in the extended care facility]." The staff and the other residents saw her determination, optimistic outlook, and lack of self-centeredness as an inspirational example to others. Jane saw herself as just doing what she has always done: being positive and making the most of what she is given.

Although the facility where she lived was 16 miles from her former town, she took a keen interest in her visitors, and many more individuals visited her than any other resident of the facility. She was forced to leave behind her former lifestyle, and she proceeded to become as fully active a participant in her new community as she was physically able, and she continued to serve others by just being herself. She had a strong faith that she was in God's care. Compared with herself at 50, she was less afraid of death, felt a greater connection to the universe, and took greater pleasure in her inner life.

Jane went from very active to below average in her activity level; from independent to needing help with bathing, dressing, and using the toilet; from vital and healthy to very sick; from living in her own household to living in an institution. Yet her lifelong approach to life provided enormous resilience, and her continuity of viewpoint and outlook triumphed over seemingly overwhelming changes in her circumstances. She is certainly a strong testimonial for the capacity of a clear and untroubled mind to prevail over illness and dependence. In our most recent interview with her, in 1997, at age 74 she was a still a confident but humble person who appreciated fully that without the help and supportive environment, she would not be able to manage. But she still took fullest advantage of all opportunities. She continued to inspire visits from staff and residents of the retirement community, but perhaps more revealing was that after four years, a steady flow of visitors from her former town still came to see her.

These cases illustrate the attractiveness of continuity as a strategy for adapting to change. Continuity is often a conscious goal, and the desire for continuity can prevail over substantial challenges. But discontinuity, even if undesired and unexpected, can be adapted to successfully, as Jane's case shows.

Inner continuity concerns the structure and evolution of the ideas and predispositions that form an important part of the enduring inner landscape of human consciousness. Considerable evidence suggests that psychobiological aspects of consciousness, such as temperament and drives, are generally consistent over time, but in advanced old age these forces are diminished gradually by physical aging. Yet no matter how diminished, enough usually remains of temperament and drives for others to see a linkage with the past self.

A considerable body of evidence supports the persistence of general personality structure over time (McCrae 1995), but there is also evidence that some aspects of personality, such as introspection (Kogan 1990) and transcendence (Tornstam 1994), evolve over time. The metaphor of growth spirals captures the process that appears to occur. Early in life, we develop the needed attitudes, values, beliefs, and mental skills to adapt to the world as we experience it. As we move into and through adulthood, we are presented with an increasingly complex social environment, which means that the frameworks of ideas with which we enter adulthood need to be expanded gradually in each life stage to include not only more information but a more integrative perspective (Wilber 1996). Each successive life stage provides experiences that are used to evolve a more inclusive perspective on life itself, and this perspective does not require a person to continue to do all of the things that contributed to that perspective but simply to remember them. Thus, a person can understand very well the value and experience of having an occupation without currently having a job.

I will not deal here with the inner workings of personality. That subject has been covered effectively elsewhere (Kogan 1990). Instead, I focus our examination of inner continuity on ideas about the self, particularly personal agency, emotional resilience, and personal goals. I also look at beliefs about the effects of retirement.

Perceptions of inner continuity depend on memory and consciousness, and therefore they are susceptible to the tendency of the human mind to be a revisionist historian; that is, we remember the past in ways that support the present (Greenwald 1980). For this reason, retrospective approaches to the study of inner continuity are not as useful as longitudinal panel data collected from the same individuals over an extended period. I use data from the Ohio Longitudinal Study of Aging and Adaptation (OLSAA) to look at continuity of ideas over a period of 20 years in a panel of adults who were age 50 and older at the start of the study.

Continuity of the Self

Nearly all of us recognize elements of ourselves that have remained consistent over time. I recently visited three older cousins of mine who knew me well when I was a teenager but had not had any contact with me for nearly 30 years. They had no difficulty whatsoever identifying who I was and in relating to me. Their general mental models of who I was and what I was like were adapted easily to include countless changes, including my career and family history. Many things had happened, but I was still basically the same Robert Atchley to them. I must say that I share their same view. Many of the basic inner patterns that constitute my unique self have remained relatively consistent even though over the years new inner perspectives have been added, and a great deal has changed in my external social circumstances.

A very large number of interview respondents over the years have told me that when they look in a mirror they cannot believe that they have grown so old. Their inner view of themselves has remained much younger. Many of them see a great similarity between their current self and a much younger self, and this perception may well be very accurate. Indeed, our longitudinal data show that a large proportion of respondents maintained consistent self-concepts over the 20 years of our study.

I begin by looking at the dynamics of several dimensions of the self over the 20-year span of our study. I look first at two dimensions of the self-concept: self-confidence and emotional resilience. I then look at self-values or personal goals. Self-concept consists of our perceptions of our personal characteristics. The extent to which we have confidence in our ability to make things happen and our perceptions of our emotional resilience in the face of life's ups and downs constitute important elements of the self-concept.

Self-Confidence

Self-confidence is at the heart of the concept of human agency. It is difficult to imagine that a person who lacked self-confidence could think that he or she had much capacity to influence the world. Self-confidence involves two important dimensions: belief in one's ability to achieve goals and the capacity to be assertive to people in general and to people in authority in particular. In the OLSAA we measured self-confidence with a six-item scale. The items and coding are shown in Table 2.1.

Descriptive Analysis

Table 2.1 also shows the distribution of responses to the self-confidence items for the 273 respondents who answered all of the self-confidence items in the 1995 survey. A large majority of responses fell on the positive end of the continuum for all items. In absolute terms, a score of 12 or less, out of a possible 24, indicates a perceived lack of self-confidence. Only 5 (0.7%) of 737 respondents to the 1975 survey had self-confidence scores of 12 or lower. Only 1 (0.4%) of 273 respondents to the 1995 survey had a self-confidence score below 12. However, within the positive range, scores are reasonably well distributed, with a range of 11 to 24, a mean of 18.5, and a standard deviation of 2.4. Thus, over all waves of the OLSAA, nearly everyone was self-confident, but the degrees of self-confidence varied considerably.

In terms of specific items, for 1995 the proportion reporting a lack of self-confidence was greatest for "I am a go-getter" (38% disagreed) followed by "I have trouble talking to people about myself" (22.6% agreed), "I can do just about anything I set my mind to" (18.6% disagreed), and "If I want some-

TABLE 2.1. Distribution of self-confidence items, 1995 ($N = 273$)

Item	Strongly Agree (%)	Agree (%)	Disagree (%)	Strongly Disagree (%)
I can do just about anything I set my mind to.	22.0	59.5	17.6	1.0
I am a go-getter.	11.4	50.5	34.9	3.1
My life seems doomed to failure.	0.7	1.0	39.5	58.9
I'm afraid to talk to people in authority.	2.0	4.7	45.5	47.8
If I want something, I go out and get it.	14.6	68.7	13.9	2.7
I have trouble talking to people about myself.	2.4	20.2	60.3	17.2

NOTE: The positive end of the continuum is underlined.

TABLE 2.2. Mean self-confidence, by survey wave, for the total panel and for 1995 respondents

	Total Panel			1995 Respondents		
Year	N	Mean	S.D.	N	Mean	S.D.
1975	737	18.98	2.4	273	19.46	2.5
1977	578	18.78	2.5	273	19.51	2.4
1979	568	18.79	2.6	273	19.56	2.4
1981	566	18.29	2.5	273	18.96	2.4
1991	405	18.90	2.6	273	19.14	2.6
1995	273	18.54	2.4	273	18.54	2.4

thing, I go out and get it" (16.6% disagreed). Over time, the proportional distribution for each self-confidence item fluctuated only slightly.

Table 2.2 shows the mean self-confidence scores for each of the six survey waves for the total panel and for those who would survive to participate in the 1995 survey. Note that the mean self-confidence scores remained very consistent over the 20-year span in both groups. However, the core panel members who would survive to complete the 1995 survey had a slightly higher mean self-confidence score at each survey wave before 1995. Note also that the standard deviations of the self-confidence scales remained relatively constant throughout the study.

These descriptive analyses show that the degree of self-confidence is variable, but there is a great deal of consistency in group proportions and group means over the six survey waves, even if we look at only those respondents who survived to complete all six surveys. However, group means and proportions do not reflect individual change or consistency; they can be the result of cancellation effects involving numerous individual ups and downs. To assess this possibility, I next look at individual patterns of response to the self-confidence items over time.

In individual patterns, the same score over the course of the study was obviously stability. *Continuity* was defined as fluctuations of no more than 1 standard deviation on either side of the baseline score, and *discontinuity* was defined as fluctuations greater than 1 standard deviation. Using these criteria, only 5 percent had the same score over the course of the entire study, 65 percent were classified as having continuity in self-confidence, and 30 percent were classified as showing discontinuity. Of the 30 percent with discontinuity, 17 percent showed a decline in self-confidence, and 13 percent showed an increase.

When we looked at individual self-confidence scale items, stability and continuity in overall self-confidence scores resulted from offsetting changes in individual items over time for 27 percent of the cases. About 8 percent of those with discontinuity (30%) also showed patterns of offsetting changes in individual items. A case example may make this point clearer. Tess had a stable self-confidence score of 17 across all waves of the study, but she increased her rating of herself as a go-getter and decreased her rating of herself as feeling comfortable talking to people in authority. This was the most common offsetting pattern: increased sense of agency but more difficulty talking to people in authority. Another common offset was feeling less able to do just about anything (usually connected with functional limitations) accompanied by *less* fear of talking to people in authority. These cases illustrate the dynamics of self-confidence that can be masked in an analysis of aggregated scores. They suggest that people who experienced aging as a gentle slope felt an increased sense of agency, but ageism may have led to more rejection and greater difficulty talking to people in authority. However, people who experienced functional limitations appropriately felt a decrease in agency, but their increased contact with service providers may have made them more comfortable talking with people in authority.

Multivariate Analysis

Typically, researchers construct multivariate models in which a number of presumed independent variables are used to predict a dependent variable. For example, in the case of self-confidence, a model could be constructed using current values on sociodemographic predictors such as age, gender, and education; self-rated health and functional capability; and activity level to predict current level of self-confidence. The selection of these predictors is based on their correlations with self-confidence or personal agency in previous research. Table 2.3 shows the results for this type of analysis conducted on the 1995 wave of the OLSAA. As expected, 1995 health, functional capability, and activity level were correlated with 1995 self-confidence, but the sociodemographic variables did not correlate significantly with current self-confidence. In earlier research (Atchley and Scala 1998), we suggested that health variables capture the effects of social structural variables such as age, gender, and education, and the effects of sociodemographic variables on health usually have already occurred by the time people are age 50, which means that we did not pick them up in the OLSAA. This suggests that the social structural effects included in the Markus and Herzog (1991) dynamic model of the self occur before middle age and have no independent effects in later adulthood. The overall predictive power of the model is modest, with an adjusted R^2 of .276, which means that knowing the values of the independent variables allows us to improve on purely chance predictions of the dependent variable by 27.6 percent.

But the model in Table 2.3 does not take advantage of our longitudinal data, which allow us to use prior values of the independent variables and thus eliminate the problem of causal order that confounds the findings in most cross-sectional regression analysis. One of the requirements for establishing causality is that the presumed cause must occur before the presumed effect, but in cross-sectional analysis we can seldom satisfy this time order requirement. We can easily presume that age, gender, and education occurred before current self-confidence, but the same cannot be said of self-rated health, functional capability, or activity level because a drop in self-confidence could conceivably lead to a negative change in self-reporting of positive health, functional capability, or activity level.

To use the longitudinal data, we can construct lagged regression models as shown in Tables 2.4 and 2.5. In these models, prior-wave variables, including prior self-confidence, are used as independent variables. Because baseline measures are the best predictor of subsequent measures for a great many variables, researchers typically do their best to eliminate the effect of continuity over time in the dependent variable in order to "uncover" relationships that would be insignificant had prior values of the dependent variable been given an equal chance to predict its current level. In other words, conventional regression analysis methods intentionally ignore continuity as a "cause" of the dependent variable. Table 2.4 shows clearly how misleading this practice can be. Without control for the initial level of self-confidence, it appears that younger age and higher activity level are significant antecedents of 1977 self-confidence, but the predictive power of these independent variables is weak ($R^2 = .123$). However, for our purposes, we are very interested

TABLE 2.3. Cross-sectional predictors of 1995 self-confidence ($N = 216$)

Predictor	Standardized Beta Coefficient
Age	−.034
Gender	.000
Education	.079
1995 Health	.271*
1995 Functioning	.176*
1995 Activity level	.214*
R^2	.276

* Beta coefficient significant at the .01 level or better.

TABLE 2.4. Lagged predictors of 1997 self-confidence with and without lagged self-confidence

1975 Predictor	1977 Self-Confidence	
	Without 1975 Self-Confidence	With 1975 Self-Confidence
Age	−.199**	−.057
Gender	.069	.003
Education	.073	.014
Health	.055	.069
Functioning	.097	.014
Activity level	.267**	.102*
Self-confidence		.617**
R^2	.123	.424
N	440	375

* Beta coefficient significant at the .05 level or better.
** Beta coefficient significant at the .001 level or better.

in the extent to which continuity exists and the magnitude of its effects. For theoretical reasons, prior self-confidence is a significant potential "cause." When we include the baseline measure of self-confidence in the regression equation, 1975 self-confidence is by far the most powerful predictor of 1977 self-confidence (beta = .617),[1] age disappears from the equation, and activity level becomes a minor factor (beta = .102) compared with continuity in self-confidence. In addition, the overall predictive power of the equation increases substantially, to an R^2 of .424.

Table 2.5 shows lagged regression analyses for all survey waves. With only a few exceptions, continuity in self-confidence completely overshadows the effects of other potential antecedents of self-confidence, and the magnitude of continuity is indicated by the high beta coefficients for prior-wave self-confidence across the board. This effect occurs for all survey intervals, and the intervals ranged from two years to ten years. Thus, continuity is indeed a major factor in explaining self-confidence over time.

No other independent variable is significant in all of the lagged regressions. Age is significant for 1981 and 1991, with older respondents less likely to have high self-confidence. The prior-wave activity level is significant for 1977 and 1981, with active respondents more likely to have high self-confidence. Prior-wave self-rated health was significant for 1979 and 1991, with respondents in very good health more likely to have high self-confidence. Functional ca-

[1] In regression analysis, beta coefficients indicate the relative power of separate independent variables as "predictors" of the dependent variable.

pability was significant only for 1995, and education was significant only for 1991. Gender is not significant in any of the regressions. To ensure that gender was indeed nonsignificant, we ran a statistical test for significant differences between regression equations (Chow 1960). Earlier studies treating gender as a dummy variable had produced misleading findings of no gender effect in regression analyses when in fact separate analyses by gender produced markedly different regression equations (Kunkel and Atchley 1996). Throughout this book, whenever gender is used in regression analysis and appears to be nonsignificant, we applied the Chow test to make sure that we were not ignoring significant gender findings.

TABLE 2.5. Lagged predictors of self-confidence, by survey wave

Predictor	Self-Confidence				
	1977	1979	1981	1991	1995
Age	−.057	−.019	−.123**	.153**	.095
Gender	.003	.002	.005	.058	.080
Education	−.014	.056	.078	.183**	.019
1975					
Health	−.069				
Functioning	−.014				
Activity	.102*				
1977					
Health		.112*			
Functioning		.066			
Activity		−.089			
1979					
Health			.049		
Functioning			.024		
Activity			.115*		
1981					
Health				.115*	
Functioning				−.083	
Activity				.021	
1991					
Health					.075
Functioning					.208**
Activity					.009
Self-confidence					
1975	.617**				
1977		.630**			
1979			.582**		
1981				.502**	
1991					.579**
Adjusted R^2	.424	.428	.426	.398	.456
N	375	284	280	234	178

* Beta coefficient significant at the .05 level or better.
** Beta coefficient significant at the .01 level or better.

TABLE 2.6. Predictors of 1995 self-confidence (*N* = 198)

Predictor	Standardized Regression Coefficient (beta)
Age	.011
Gender	.095
Education	.026
1995	
Health	.190*
Functioning	.167*
Activity level	.030
1991 Self-confidence	.536**
R^2	.576

* Beta coefficient significant at the .05 level or better.
** Beta coefficient significant at the .01 level or better.

There is no general pattern in which any of the independent variables other than prior-wave self-confidence is a typical predictor of current self-confidence; and even when these other variables are significant, the beta coefficients for them are very modest, especially compared with prior-wave self-confidence.

To assess the relative power of continuity compared with current conditions, we performed a regression analysis that included prior self-confidence and current health, functional capability, and activity level. Table 2.6 shows the results of this analysis. Prior self-confidence remains by far the strongest predictor of current self-confidence, but current health and functional capability make a significant contribution to predicting current self-confidence, raising the overall adjusted R^2 to a relatively high .576.

The results of these various analyses look at continuity from a variety of methodological perspectives and show very clearly that continuity was by far the most common pattern with regard to self-confidence over time. Later I look at the effects of life changes such as retirement, widowhood, and disability on self-confidence, and again we find that a pattern of continuity in self-confidence is the prevalent outcome even for those who develop disability.

Emotional Resilience

Emotional resilience is a perceived capacity to deal with the emotions that can arise from the ups and downs of life. Resilience was measured in the OLSAA by an eight-item scale (shown in Table 2.7). The scale is a subset of the Philadelphia Geriatric Center (PGC) Morale Scale items that deal with

TABLE 2.7. Distribution of emotional resilience items, 1995 (*N* = 292)

Item	Strongly Agree (%)	Agree (%)	Disagree (%)	Strongly Disagree (%)
Things keep getting worse as I get older.	2.1	22.9	40.1	34.9
Little things bother me more this year.	1.7	27.1	51.2	19.9
Sometimes I think life is not worth living.	0.03	8.4	31.0	60.3
I am as happy now as when I was younger.	19.2	54.8	23.3	2.7
I have a lot to be sad about.	1.4	5.4	46.9	46.3
I am afraid of a lot of things.	0.03	6.2	46.9	46.6
I get mad more than I used to.		12.9	48.6	38.4
I take things hard.	0.7	18.5	48.6	32.2

NOTE: The positive end of the continuum is underlined.

the respondent's perceived need to cope with emotions such as irritability, sadness, anger, or fear and to maintain happiness and avoid hopelessness.

Descriptive Analysis

Once again, nearly all respondents were in the positive region of emotional resilience. Emotional resilience scale scores theoretically ranged from 8 to 32, with 16 or lower being in the negative region of the scale conceptually. Only three of the 1995 respondents (1.1% of 270) scored 16, and none scored lower. However, within the positive range of emotional resilience, the respondents were well distributed, with a 1995 range of 16 to 32, a mean of 25.7, and a standard deviation of 3.9. This pattern occurred for all waves of the survey.

The means for emotional resilience were quite consistent across the various survey waves (for specific data, see Table A.1.). Fluctuations in means and standard deviations were minor, although the panel members who would survive to complete the 1995 survey had slightly higher mean emotional resilience than the total panel for each wave from 1975 through 1991.

In terms of individual items, the greatest proportion reported negative experience for "Little things bother me more this year" (28.8% agreed), followed by "I am as happy now as when I was younger" (26% disagreed), "Things keep getting worse as I get older" (25% agreed), and "I take things hard" (19.2% agreed). Thus, the total scores masked some negative responses because they were offset by strongly positive responses on other items, such as those about hopelessness, sadness, and fear. To explore this pattern of offsetting responses, I now look at individual patterns for individual emotional resilience items.

We expected that the emotional resilience scale would be more sensitive to current mood and therefore might show less prevalence of continuity over time for individuals. This turned out to be the case. When we examined patterns over time in emotional resilience for individuals, 4 percent were stable, 50 percent showed continuity, and 46 percent showed discontinuity — 26 percent with a substantial decline and 20 percent with a substantial improvement. About one third of the cases of stability and continuity involved a pattern of increases offsetting declines, and 9 percent among the 20 percent of cases showing an overall increase over time involved increases outweighing decreases for specific emotional resilience items. On the other hand, only 3 percent of the 26 percent who showed a decline had offsetting increases. Interestingly, the specific items most likely to account for change were the same for both patterns of increase and decrease in emotional resilience: "Little things bother me more this year," "I take things hard," and "I get mad more than I used to."

Thus, the pattern of consistent mean emotional resilience over time involved a substantial proportion of offsetting individual patterns of increase and decrease. In addition, individual patterns of both continuity and discontinuity often involved offsetting increases and decreases.

Multivariate Analysis

As we learned in the previous section on self-confidence, it is important to look at previous scores on self-rated health, functional capability, activity level, and emotional resilience as lagged predictors of current emotional resilience for each survey wave. Table 2.8 shows that previous levels of emotional resilience are by far the best predictors of current emotional resilience. However, lagged effects of previous self-rated health are significant in the equations for 1977, 1991, and 1995; education is significant for 1977; age is significant in the equation for 1981; and activity level is significant in the equation for 1979. Gender is not significant in any of the regressions. However, the beta coefficients for these variables were modest, especially compared with prior-level emotional resilience. Only prior-wave self-rated health showed a persistent relationship with emotional resilience, with very good prior-wave health being a significant predictor of high emotional resilience in three of the five regression equations.

When we look at the combination of prior emotional resilience and current sociodemographic, health, and activity variables, prior emotional resilience is by far the most influential factor in the equation (beta = .550)

TABLE 2.8. Lagged predictors of emotional resilience, by survey wave

Predictor	Dependent Variable: Emotional Resilience				
	1977	1979	1981	1991	1995
Age	−.064	−.016	−.149**	.098	−.001
Gender	.021	.014	.022	.084	.035
Education	.114*	.022	.041	.065	.021
1975					
Health	.163**				
Functioning	.074				
Activity	.058				
1977					
Health		.077			
Functioning		.067			
Activity		.134**			
1979					
Health			.080		
Functioning			.043		
Activity			.044		
1981					
Health				.163**	
Functioning				.071	
Activity				.013	
1991					
Health					.193**
Functioning					.052
Activity					.014
Emotional resilience					
1975	.512**				
1977		.627**			
1979			.661**		
1981				.501**	
1991					.580**
Adjusted R^2	.393	.450	.474	.311	.459
N	511	394	351	229	171

 * Beta coefficient significant at the .05 level or better.
 ** Beta coefficient significant at the .01 level or better.

followed by current self-rated health (.197) and current activity level (.145). These three variables account for slightly more than 50 percent of the variation in emotional resilience in 1995 (for specific data, see Table A.2.).

Again, through a series of descriptive and multivariate causal analyses we see that continuity of emotional resilience is the dominant pattern, but for emotional resilience there is more deviation away from continuity than was true for self-confidence.

Personal Goals

People enact their self-reflective values through their structure of personal goals. In the OLSAA, personal goals were assessed by asking respondents to attach a degree of importance to each of 16 personal goals listed in Table 2.9. The table also shows the distribution of importance attached to each item in the 1995 survey.

Descriptive Analysis

A striking finding in Table 2.9 that, as we shall see, applies to all waves of the study, is that very few of the goals listed were considered unimportant. But the fact that more than 50 percent of the respondents thought that being prominent in community affairs and being accepted by influential people were unimportant supports the observation made many years ago by Clark and Anderson (1967) that after middle age, people tend to gravitate away from values that drive the economic and social hierarchies within the community and move instead toward "secondary" values such as family ties and personal qualities like being dependable, self-reliant, and self-accepting. These were precisely the personal goals deemed "very important" by a majority of the 1995 respondents, all of whom were 70 or older.

The individual personal goals items were summed for each survey wave

TABLE 2.9. Importance attached to selected personal goals, 1995 (*N* = 307)

	Very Important (%)	Important (%)	Unimportant (%)	Very Unimportant (%)
Being well read and informed	50.0	48.3	1.7	
Having close ties with my family	75.3	23.0	1.3	0.3
Being prominent in community affairs	2.4	20.1	57.4	20.1
Having a substantial family income	27.1	66.2	6.7	
Having a satisfying job	28.8	37.6	17.6	16.0
Forming close, long-lasting friendships	43.0	51.7	4.6	0.7
Being self-reliant	61.4	34.6	1.3	
Seeking new experiences	20.5	58.1	19.1	2.3
Having a comfortable place to live	56.4	43.0	0.3	0.3
Having roots in the community	29.7	55.7	12.3	2.3
Being seen as a good person by others	39.5	52.6	6.9	1.0
Being dependable and reliable	71.1	28.2	0.3	0.3
Being accepted by influential people	5.7	30.0	52.2	12.1
Having a close, intimate relationship with another person	43.1	42.7	12.9	
Being a religious person	27.2	47.7	16.6	1.4
Being able to accept myself as I am	58.3	41.0	0.7	8.6

to provide a measure of goal directedness, the extent to which the respondents thought that many goals were important. There is little variation in mean goal directedness scores over the course of the study, either for the panel as a whole or for the respondents who would remain in the study to answer all of the personal goals items in 1995 (for specific data, see Table A.3.). Very important goals were given a score of 1 and very unimportant goals a score of 4. Thus, lower personal goals scores indicate a greater number of goals rated very important or important. Theoretically, the minimum score was 16, and the maximum was 64. In reality, scores ranged from 16 to 52. The mean of means across all waves was 28.25, which reflects that most people in the panel had a large number of goals they felt were important or very important.

As might be expected, personal goals were more stable over time compared with self-confidence and emotional resilience. Stability and continuity accounted for 79 percent of cases, and 21 percent showed discontinuity in goal directedness—11 percent showed an increase, and 10 percent showed a decrease. Offsetting increases and decreases occurred in about one quarter of the cases of stability or continuity, but only about 10 percent of the discontinuity cases involved offsetting increases and decreases.

Not surprisingly, the importance attached to having a satisfying job was the personal goal by far the most likely to be downgraded because most respondents retired during the study. However, even among those who were retired, having had a satisfying job remained an important goal for 70 percent. Another personal goal likely to decline in importance was being prominent in the community. Goals that were likely to increase in importance included forming long-lasting friendships and having a close, intimate relationship with another person.

Multivariate Analysis

Table 2.10 shows the 1975 predictors of personal goal directedness in 1977, both with and without the 1975 personal goals scores. Without 1975 personal goals, only activity level was related to 1977 personal goals, with respondents having lower activity levels also having fewer important personal goals. The predictive value of this equation was poor, with an R^2 of just .064. However, when 1975 personal goals scores were included in the equation, the continuity of personal goals was by far the more powerful predictor (beta = .526), and the R^2 increased to a modest .321. The point here is that without measures of the continuity of personal goals, current personal goals remain a

TABLE 2.10. Lagged predictors of 1977 personal goals with and without 1975 personal goals ($N = 516$)

1975	1977 Personal Goals (%)	
	Without 1975 Personal Goals	With 1975 Personal Goals
Age	−.047	−.034
Sex	.021	.016
Gender	.075	.038
Health	.022	.032
Functioning	.025	.035
Activity	−.122**	−.119*
Personal goal		.526**
Adjusted R^2	.064	.321

* Beta coefficient significant at the .05 level or better.
** Beta coefficient significant at the .01 level or better.

mystery because they are not strongly related to either sociodemographic or situational variables.

When we look at the time-lagged regression analysis in Table 2.11, we see that for personal goals, continuity is an even stronger force than was true for the preceding measures of internal continuity. Only activity level for 1977, 1979, and 1995 contributes to the prediction of personal goals independent of the effects of continuity over time in personal goals, and the regression coefficients for activity level are modest. However, using previous levels of personal goal directedness, continuity over time allows us to predict an increasingly larger proportion of the variation in personal goals scores.

Adding in current health and activity improves the prediction of personal goals, as Table 2.12 shows. 1995 functional capability and activity level do make significant contributions to the equation, but the overall predictive capability of this analysis is not much better than that achieved by the time-lagged analysis shown in Table 2.11.

Personal goals were extremely stable over time in all of our analyses. However, even a variable with such a high prevalence of continuity showed significant relationships with current functional capability and activity level.

Beliefs about the Effects of Retirement

Thus far, I have looked at self-perceptions and self-referent values. In this section, I look at continuity over time in beliefs. Beliefs are ideas about what is true of the world around us. Some beliefs are based on our experiences, but

TABLE 2.11. Lagged predictors of personal goals, by survey wave

Predictor	Personal Goals				
	1977	1979	1981	1991	1995
Age	−.034	.011	.022	.077	.029
Gender	.014	.013	.063	.023	.075
Education	.034	.014	−.006	−.008	.018
1975					
Health	.022				
Functioning	.018				
Activity	−.117*				
1977					
Health		−.038			
Functioning		−.015			
Activity		−.116*			
1979					
Health			−.022		
Functioning			−.007		
Activity			−.036		
1981					
Health				−.080	
Functioning				−.009	
Activity				−.108	
1991					
Health					.030
Functioning					.000
Activity					−.136*
Personal goals					
1975	.525**				
1977		.527**			
1979			.653**		
1981				.605**	
1991					.565**
Adjusted R^2	.321	.316	.365	.359	.386
N	557	434	370	201	154

 * Beta coefficient significant at the .05 level or better.
** Beta coefficient significant at the .01 level or better.

many are simply ideas we receive as part of our socialization and accept on faith with no feeling of a need to test their accuracy.

Descriptive Analysis

We asked the OLSAA respondents to tell us the extent to which they attributed the beliefs listed in Table 2.13 to retired people in general. As the table shows, the respondents generally believed that retirement seldom had negative effects on physical health, premature mortality, mental health, aging, adjustment, social relationships, or social activities. However,

TABLE 2.12. Selected predictors of 1995 personal goals ($N = 124$)

Predictor	Standardized Regression Coefficient (beta)
Age	.030
Gender	.091
Education	.079
1995	
Health	.082
Functioning	.150*
Activity	−.305**
Personal goals	
1981	.377*
1991	.307**
R^2	.522

* Beta coefficient significant at the .05 level or better.
** Beta coefficient significant at the .01 level or better.

TABLE 2.13. Beliefs about retirement, 1995 ($N = 298$)

Belief	Extent to Which Statements Apply to Retired People in General (%)			
	Almost None	A Few	Many	Almost All
Retirement causes people to get sick.	26.2	65.1	8.4	0.3
Retirement leads to premature death.	37.1	55.8	6.8	0.3
When people retire, they miss their jobs.	5.0	48.5	42.2	4.3
When people retire, they lose touch with who they are.	28.9	58.7	12.4	
Retirement causes people to age more rapidly.	27.1	59.5	13.4	
Retirement is a difficult adjustment for most people.	12.3	52.5	31.2	4.0
Retirement causes people to suffer mental problems.	37.4	57.4	5.3	
Retired people have trouble finding things to do.	17.5	56.5	25.2	0.7
When people retire, they lose touch with their friends.	25.4	55.8	17.5	1.3

many respondents believed that a substantial number of retired people miss their jobs.

The individual beliefs about retirement were summed to provide an overall score of the extent to which respondents accepted the idea that negative effects of retirement were widespread. The scale has a theoretical minimum of 8 and a maximum of 32; in actuality the minimum was 10, and the maximum was 31. Scores for 1995 are distributed normally, and the mean of 17.6 indicates that respondents believe that most of the stereotypes about retirement apply to only a few people.

Over time the panel became significantly less likely to believe that negative stereotypes about retirement were widely applicable. This was true both for the panel as a whole and for those who remained in the study throughout it (for specific data, see Table A.4.).

Multivariate Analysis

Because we might expect those who are retired to have a different perspective on beliefs about retirement compared with those with no personal experience of it, we included retirement status as part of our regression analysis of retirement beliefs.

Table 2.14 shows that activity level is the only significant time-lagged predictor of retirement beliefs in 1979, with those who were less active being more likely to accept negative beliefs about retirement. However, the predictive power of this equation is trivial ($R^2 = .028$). Continuity of retirement beliefs adds significantly to the equation (beta = .605), and the R^2 increases to .390. Once again, we find that by themselves, sociodemographic, health, and social situational variables are poorly related to interindividual differences in ideas over time.

Table 2.15 shows the time-lagged effects of age, self-rated health, functional capability, activity level, retirement status, and retirement beliefs on retirement beliefs in subsequent waves, from 1979 to 1995. As in the previous analyses, continuity in retirement beliefs is by far the most powerful factor in understanding the dynamics of retirement beliefs over time. Interestingly, experiencing retirement had no effect on respondents' beliefs about retired people in general.

TABLE 2.14. Lagged predictors of 1979 beliefs about retirement with and without 1977 retirement beliefs ($N = 478$)

	1979 Beliefs about Retirement	
1977 Predictor	Without 1977 Beliefs	With 1977 Beliefs
Age	−.082	−.031
Gender	.069	.069
Education	.067	.047
Health	−.049	−.038
Functioning	−.047	−.046
Activity level	−.173**	−.112*
Retirement status	−.051	−.058
Retirement beliefs		.605**
R^2	.028	.390

* Beta coefficient significant at the .05 level or better.
** Beta coefficient significant at the .01 level or better.

TABLE 2.15. Lagged predictors of retirement beliefs, by survey wave

Predictor	Retirement Beliefs			
	1979	1981	1991	1995
Age	−.022	−.002	.025	−.032
Gender	.076*	.046	.007	.037
Education	.051	.022	−.130**	.054
1977				
Health	−.030			
Functioning	−.062			
Activity	−.109*			
Retirement status	−.057			
1979				
Health		−.058		
Functioning		−.066		
Activity		−.047		
Retirement status		−.031		
1981				
Health			−.027	
Functioning			−.072	
Activity			.003	
Retirement status			−.048	
1991				
Health				−.019
Functioning				.049
Activity				−.065
Retirement status				−.030
Retirement beliefs				
1977	.606**			
1979		.535**		
1981			.548**	
1991				.680**
Adjusted R^2	.400	.285	.308	.460
N	420	397	244	188

* Beta coefficient significant at the .05 level or better.
** Beta coefficient significant at the .01 level or better.

Summary

The data reported in this chapter show very clearly that continuity over time is the most prevalent pattern for all of the inner constructs we examined: self-confidence, emotional resilience, personal goals, and beliefs about retirement. The only variable that showed change over time was retirement beliefs, where the panel became significantly less likely to accept negative stereotypes about retirement over the course of the study. Interestingly, this change was unrelated to retirement status or age, which suggests that stereotypes about retirement may be becoming less negative in the general population.

Regardless of the type of data analysis used, stability and continuity emerged as dominant patterns. But these findings do not mean that continuity was uniform or ubiquitous. In all of the analyses, there was wide variability across individuals in baseline measures of each mental construct we examined. In addition, although the regression analyses generally produced quite large adjusted R^2 statistics, much variation remained unexplained.

Age seldom had predictive value when the effects of other variables were controlled. This makes sense if we expect that people will maintain their inner frameworks of ideas as they age.

Some readers might be puzzled that the sociodemographic variables of gender and education, which have been found to be so important in explaining so many variables in gerontology, were of so little value in our analyses of inner continuity. My best guess as to why this occurred involves two factors. First, the effects of gender and education on self-confidence, emotional resilience, personal goals, or retirement beliefs may well have occurred long before we began to study our panel, who were all age 50 or older when our study began. Second, gender and education may have indirect effects on mental constructs through their relationships to self-rated health, functional capability, and activity levels. In the OLSAA, gender and education were highly correlated with all three variables. Women and respondents with lower education reported lower self-rated health, functional capability, and activity levels.

Health variables had surprisingly little effect on mental constructs when continuity of mental constructs was factored into the equation. Only emotional resilience showed a time-lagged relationship with prior self-rated health in several regression equations. All of the other relationships of self-rated health or functional capability involved the relationship of current health to current mental constructs. These data suggest that structures of ideas are resistant to the influence of health changes, except when they involve severe disability.

Activity level had a sporadic but persistent relationship to inner structures. For each of the four inner structures we examined, the previous activity level was a predictor of current inner structure for at least one of the survey intervals. Although certainly not a strong finding, this discovery suggests some support for the idea that more active people are more capable of maintaining continuity in their inner structures of ideas.

3 | External Continuity

External continuity occurs in the social arrangements people create to meet their needs. Lifestyle visions and social opportunities are the main forces influencing the types of social arrangements people create and to which they aspire. For people who plan ahead, there are two ways of constructing an overview of the type of life they want. The first view emphasizes opportunities, and lifestyle decisions involve choosing from a set of positively valued alternatives. The second view emphasizes constraints, and people attempt to construct the most positive lifestyle possible given their social or cultural limitations. Of course, there are people who approach life from a fatalistic viewpoint in which they see themselves as being at the mercy of economic and social forces and having little choice but to make the best of whatever circumstances come their way. But even this last scenario usually results in a life routine that people become motivated to preserve because it becomes their customary way of adapting.

From midlife on, lifestyles usually represent the maintenance and continuation of patterns that were constructed gradually over a period of many years. But because they address basic needs for food, clothing, shelter, and companionship, these lifestyles represent metastructures that can support changes in values. For example, people in later life often report that over time their inner life and contemplative spirituality become more important to them. This change is usually an increase in the degree of importance attached to a particular type of life experience rather than a new interest. This increasing interest in contemplative spirituality can be supported by a lifestyle that represents a social "automatic pilot" that routinely handles their basic needs, and the individual is freer to concentrate attention on contemplative aspects of life. Indeed, older people can come to see external continuity as even more important than earlier in life because in later life external continuity provides a basis for social security; it provides a stable platform for venturing forth into

new inner territory. Of course, basic lifestyle patterns can also serve as a platform for moving into new social territory, too.

In this chapter I look at evidence for continuity in lifestyles over time in middle age and later life. Because I am most interested in long-term patterns of external continuity, I look primarily at data for the 308 Ohio Longitudinal Study of Aging and Adaptation (OLSAA) respondents who responded to five or six survey waves, including the 1995 survey. Dimensions of lifestyle I consider first include living arrangements, household composition, marital status, income adequacy, and primary modes of transportation. Decisions about living arrangements, marriage, childrearing, and household routines have important implications for the type of specific dwelling people choose. People adapt *to* their physical environments and also reshape these environments to enhance personal or household functioning and life satisfaction. Thus, remaining in the same household can be an important aspect of external continuity. However, lifestyle activities are the major focus of our analysis. After all, lifestyle activities are an important resource that people use in their attempts to adapt and to create an experience of life satisfaction. Lifestyle activities include productive ones such as employment, household work, or volunteer service; social activities such as spending time with friends and family; physical activities such as gardening or sports; organizational activities such as participating in professional organizations or churches; and individual activities such as hobbies or reading. Note that most of the types of activities I consider occur in a context shaped by groups and social roles. I begin with a discussion of living arrangements, household composition, and marital status.

Living Arrangements, Household Composition, and Marital Status

Living arrangements comprise the type of dwelling a person occupies and whether that person lives alone or with other people. If a person lives with other people, we also want to know the nature of the person's relationship to others in the household.

When our study began in 1975, none of our respondents lived in group quarters such as nursing homes, group homes, or assisted living. They all lived in independent households, and more than 80 percent owned their homes. By 1995, nearly all were still living in independent households, although some of these households were located in continuing care retirement

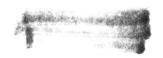

TABLE 3.1. Living arrangements, by residential mobility status (*N* = 302)

Living Arrangements	Moved		Did Not Move		% Moved
	N	%	*N*	%	
Alone throughout	12	11.3	31	15.8	27.9
Couple					
Only	36	34.0	82	41.8	30.5
+ Others	17	16.0	49	25.0	25.8
Couple to others	8	7.5	9	4.6	47.1
Couple to alone	28	26.4	24	12.2	53.8
Alone to couple					
Remarriage	5	4.7	1	0.5	83.3
Total	106	99.9	196	99.9	35.1
Mean age	78.1		76.8		
Median age	77.0		75.0		

communities. Persons who moved to nursing homes tended to be lost to follow-up for two reasons: most were single individuals, and mail was not forwarded to them after six months, or most of those that we did locate were cognitively impaired and could not respond to our interview. Of the 308 respondents to the 1995 survey, only two lived in nursing homes.

More than 60 percent of the 308 long-term respondents lived in the same dwelling over the entire study period. We do not know whether moving was voluntary or involuntary, but by comparing those who moved with those who did not, we begin to see a picture of how changes in marital status and household composition can combine to influence changes in residence.

Table 3.1 shows various types of living arrangements and changes in living arrangements for the minority who moved during the study and the majority who did not. Movers were substantially less likely to live in an intact marital situation: 66.8 percent of the stayers were in intact couples throughout the study, but only 50 percent of the movers were in intact couples. It was change in marital status that most influenced moving, not just living alone. Of the 184 respondents who remained part of a married couple throughout the study, only 28.8 percent moved. Among the 43 respondents who lived alone throughout the study, only 27.9 percent moved.

However, among those who changed from living in a married couple to living alone, a majority (53.8%) moved. One quarter of the movers consisted of those who became widowed during the study, nearly all of whom were women. Of widows who shifted from living as part of a couple to living with others, about half took new people into their customary dwelling and thus did not move, and about half moved into a different dwelling that they shared with others. Most of those who moved into a different dwelling did not live with adult children but instead lived with other relatives or unrelated adults. On the other hand, two thirds of widows who stayed in their customary dwellings and lived with others shared their households with an adult daughter. About 5 percent of the movers did so in connection with marriage or remarriage. Only one stayer remarried.

Of those who moved, 61.3 percent made no change in their household composition; they moved as a couple, family, or individual living alone. By comparison, 82.6 percent of those who did not move experienced stability of their household composition. Only 13.6 percent of the total 1995 panel experienced a change in both household composition and residence. In their totality, these data confirm that continuity over time in both household composition and dwelling is very common indeed.

Income Adequacy

An important part of the potential for continuity in lifestyle rests on having the income required to support that lifestyle. In each survey wave, respondents were asked to answer "yes" or "no" to the question, "Do you consider your present family or household income enough to meet your living expenses?" Even though there was considerable income diversity in the panel, 85.1 percent reported that their income was adequate to support their customary lifestyle throughout the study. Another 5.5 percent reported that their income went from inadequate to adequate over the 20-year course of the study. Inadequate income throughout the study was reported by 2.6 percent. Of the 6.8 percent who reported negative fluctuations in income adequacy, 2.3 percent reported a decline, and 4.5 percent reported several ups and downs in income adequacy and were classified as precarious.

Women represented 59 percent of the 1995 respondents, but among those who had inadequate incomes throughout the study or who experienced inadequate income at some point during the study, women represented 75.9 percent. Divorce was a primary cause of long-term income problems for both men and women, as was widowhood for women. Only two married respondents had inadequate incomes throughout. Loss of income adequacy and precarious income adequacy were both concentrated among widows.

As a whole, these data show that continuity or improvement in income adequacy was the perception reported by more than 90 percent of the 1995 respondents. Thus, the financial underpinnings needed for continuity in lifestyles were present for a very large majority of the long-term respondents.

Modes of Transportation

In the community studied, there is no public transportation — neither buses nor taxicabs. However, the local senior center operates a transportation service that elders or disabled individuals can use to get out into the community for shopping, health care, and community events. But, as in most small towns in the United States, most people rely on private automobiles. Thus, for most people, continuing to be able to drive is a major support for lifestyle continuity.

Fortunately for them, 83.7 percent of respondents continued to be able to drive throughout the study. However, 11.7 percent drove at one time but no longer do. About 60 percent of the 36 respondents who no longer drive are now passengers in cars driven by their spouses or someone else. About one quarter use the senior center transportation service. Interestingly, five respondents (1.6%) became drivers during the study and still drive. A small number cited walking as their primary means of transportation at one time or another in the study, but only one cited walking on all six surveys. Our major point here is that most of the respondents were able to continue their customary means of transportation throughout the study.

We have found that in terms of living arrangements, household composition, income adequacy, and means of transportation, continuity is by far the most prevalent pattern in these external structures of lifestyle. Now I turn our attention to patterns of activity, the heart of lifestyle.

Patterns of Activity: Stability, Continuity, and Change over Time

First, I look at a lagged regression analysis of overall activity level, similar to the analyses of continuity in the internal measures examined in the previous chapter. Table 3.2 shows that activity level is quite predictable from wave to wave of the OLSAA, with four out of of five R^2 statistics greater than .64 and previous activity levels contributing the most to the regression equations. However, there are some interesting differences in predictors across the various survey intervals.

Although 1975 activity level was the prime predictor of 1977 activity level, age, gender, and 1975 self-confidence also contributed significantly to explaining the variation in 1977 activity level. Predictors of 1979 activity level were 1977 activity level, 1977 self-confidence, and 1977 self-rated health scores. As predictors of 1981 activity level, only previous activity levels, gen-

TABLE 3.2. Lagged predictors of activity level, by survey wave

Predictor	Activity Level				
	1977	1979	1981	1991	1995
Age	−.107**	−.025	−.049	−.203**	−.102*
Gender	.071**	.011	.099**	.123**	.004
Education	.018	.006	.131**	.045	.031
1975					
Confidence	.097**				
Health	.055				
Functioning	.024				
1977					
Confidence		.097**			
Health		.074*			
Functioning		.018			
1979					
Confidence			.067		
Health			.021		
Functioning			.031		
1981					
Confidence				.019	
Health				.094*	
Functioning				.008	
1991					
Confidence					.041
Health					.151**
Functioning					.009
Activity level					
1975	.766**				
1977		.761**			
1979			.717**		
1981				.612**	
1991					.780**
Adjusted R^2	.690	.663	.611	.494	.673
N	462	346	322	253	212

 * Beta coefficient significant at the .05 level or better.
** Beta coefficient significant at the .001 level or better.

der, and education were significant. Predictors of 1991 activity level were 1981 activity level, age, gender, and 1981 self-rated health. By 1995, the significant predictors of activity level were 1991 activity level, age, and 1991 self-rated health.

Self-confidence was a persistent predictor of activity level, being significant for the two initial intervals examined. Independent of previous activity levels, self-confidence was an important determinant of activity level. It is important to remember that these are lagged regressions in which the causal order of the independent variables is not in question. Thus, high self-confidence was an independent cause of high activity level later for the intervals when the panel was youngest. This makes sense; a high level of self-confidence is probably a prerequisite for a high activity level. In addition, previous good health was a significant independent predictor of activity level for 1991 and 1995. This suggests that as the panel aged, health constrained activities.

Age was a significant predictor of activity level for three of the intervals, with older age being associated with a lower activity level. But this was true only for women. When separate regressions were run for men and women, age was never a significant predictor of activity level for men. Why is age significant for women but not for men? Gender differences in health or physical functioning cannot be the reason because the effects of these variables were controlled in the analysis. A more likely explanation is that the age dispersion is greater for women than for men. For example, even at baseline in 1975 the proportion of women who were age 75 or older was significantly higher (18.9%) than for men (14.1%). By 1991, 30.6 percent of women were age 80 or older compared with 22.3 percent of men. Thus, aging causes activity level to go down, independent of the effects of changes in health or physical functioning or self-confidence; and because more women are exposed to this risk, age is a predictor of future activity levels for women but not for men.

These results show that there is considerable continuity over time in overall activity level. But what about the patterns over time for the various types of activity that go together to make up a respondent's overall activity level? Next I turn to an analysis of types of lifestyle activity and how they changed over time in the OLSAA.

Data from the OLSAA can also be used to examine continuity and discontinuity in the patterns that make up lifestyle. These data come mostly from responses to a series of 18 items asking respondents to report the frequency with which they participated in various types of activity. These activity types were general categories of activity, such as participation in civic organizations, rather than specific activities such as participation in the Kiwanis Club. Using factor analysis, we were able to cluster these general types of activity into even more abstract categories: activities involving socializing, requiring physical capability, and involving participation in organizations; being with family; and hobbies and solitary activities such as reading. These more abstract categories, the 18 general categories, and the 1975 distribution of OLSAA panel members on each activity type are shown in Table 3.3. In terms of socializing, being with children and grandchildren and being with friends were lifestyle keystones for a majority of respondents (60 to 63% of 1975 respondents said they engaged in these activities often or very often). Among activities involving physical capability, gardening was the most common (63% reported gardening often or very often). Attending church functions was the most

TABLE 3.3. Distribution of activity frequencies, 1975 ($N = 1,174$)

	Very Often 6	Often 5	Sometimes 4	Seldom 3	Very Seldom 2	Never 1	Missing	Often or Very Often/Never
Socializing								
Spectator art	7.2	18.7	37.1	13.7	12.9	10.3	206	25.9/10.3
Participating in games	7.4	17.3	27.2	11.4	17.5	19.1	205	24.7/19.1
Being with friends	13.3	47.5	32.0	4.1	2.9	0.2	189	60.8/0.2
Attending social gatherings	3.8	16.6	43.0	17.0	13.0	6.6	196	20.4/6.6
Physical activity								
Gardening	33.4	29.4	22.2	5.7	4.8	4.5	195	62.8/4.5
Participating in sports	8.4	13.2	19.6	12.1	15.4	31.2	222	21.6/31.2
Attending sports events	7.3	15.6	28.3	9.8	18.2	20.8	215	22.9/20.8
Travel	13.8	35.1	34.7	6.5	6.7	3.3	193	48.9/3.3
Organizations								
Politics (not voting)	9.9	21.4	24.4	13.0	12.0	19.3	202	33.1/19.3
Occupational organizations	4.2	11.9	18.1	9.7	13.4	42.7	225	16.1/42.7
Service organizations	5.6	15.1	22.8	10.0	13.7	32.8	216	20.7/32.8
Attending church functions	17.4	20.7	25.3	11.8	13.0	11.7	198	38.1/11.7
Family: being with children and grandchildren	22.9	39.8	24.7	4.1	4.7	3.8	236	62.7/3.8
Hobbies								
Participatory art	7.0	10.2	16.2	11.8	17.7	37.1	225	17.2/37.1
Handiwork	18.6	19.9	25.3	9.5	10.8	15.9	207	38.5/15.9
Collecting	5.1	10.5	20.8	11.2	18.0	34.3	222	31.3/34.3
Reading and TV								
Reading	35.6	38.0	18.8	4.1	2.3	1.1	192	73.6/1.1
TV	24.8	48.0	22.6	3.1	1.3	0.1	185	72.0/0.1

common form of organizational participation (38% often or very often) followed by involvement in political organizations (33% often or very often) and civic organizations (21% often or very often). The hobbies most commonly done often or very often were handiwork (38%) and collecting (31%). Note that compared with socializing and gardening, high organizational participation and high participation in hobbies were much less prevalent. On the other hand, the usually solitary activity of reading, over which participants potentially had the most control, was done often or very often by 74 percent of respondents.

Activities varied a great deal in terms of the proportion of elders who said they *never* participated in them. The proportion who said they never socialized with friends was negligible (0.2%) as was the proportion who never spent time with children or grandchildren (3.8%). However, the proportion never participating was much higher for occupation-based organizations such as unions or professional associations (42.7%)[1] and voluntary organizations (32.8%), for hobbies such as collecting (34.3%), or for involvement in art or music (37.1%).

I turn next to a discussion of overall activity levels and changes in them over the 20-year span of the study. Then I move to a detailed examination of patterns of continuity and discontinuity for being with children and grandchildren, being with friends, gardening, attending church functions, participating in civic organizations, doing handiwork, collecting, and reading. These analyses show that summary measures of activity level and participation in various activity categories changed only modestly over the course of the study for respondents who participated for the duration of the study. But because of cancellation effects, patterns in which increases are offset by declines, summary measures often masked much greater intraindividual fluctuations and interindividual differences over time.

When the 18 activity items are summed into an overall activity level, the resulting actual scale scores range from a low of 25 to a high of 101. (The theoretical minimum and maximum are 18 and 108, respectively.) This scale is distributed normally with a mean of means across all six surveys of 65.9 and a mean standard deviation of 10. Most of the respondents were relatively active people throughout the study. As Table 3.4 shows, compared with the total panel, those who would remain in the panel to respond in 1995 had a slightly higher activity level at each data point. For the 1995 respondents, there was a modest decline in the mean activity level from 69.8 in 1975 to

[1] This was true even before retirement for respondents who were employed in 1975.

TABLE 3.4. Mean activity level for 1995 respondents and for the total panel, 1975 to 1995

	1975	1977	1979	1981	1991	1995
1995 respondents (N = 308)	69.8	67.4	66.0	66.3	64.3	61.8
Total panel	66.5	62.61	62.7	62.9	62.9	61.8
N	920	772	624	625	405	308

TABLE 3.5. Patterns of overall activity level, 1975 to 1995

Pattern	N	%[a]
Consistent	152	50.7
Increase	8	2.7
Decrease		
Total	113	37.6
−1 S.D. 67		
−2 S.D. 33		
−3 S.D. 13		
U shape	11	3.7
Inverted U	11	3.7
Omitted	5	1.7
Total	300	100.1

[a] Rows do not add to 100.0 percent because of rounding.

61.8 in 1995. However, this modest drop in the mean activity level is a mirage because it combines offsetting patterns.

To look at individual patterns of change in overall activity level over the six waves of the OLSAA, we examined each of the 308 individuals' patterns of scores over time. We categorized these patterns into five basic ones: continuity,[2] increase, decrease, U-shaped, and inverted U-shaped. An "other" category was also provided for five cases that did not fit into one of the basic patterns. Table 3.5 shows the distribution of cases by pattern. More than half (50.7%) of the 1995 respondents showed a pattern of continuity, which was defined operationally as fluctuations of less than 1 standard deviation from their beginning score (the mean standard deviation was about 10 scale points). A small number (2.7%) experienced an increase in activity level (increase greater than 1 standard deviation from their initial score); and 37.6 percent reported a decrease greater than 1 standard deviation. Among those who reported a decrease, 13 reported decreases of more than 3 standard deviations from their initial scores, and 33 reported decreases of more than 2 standard

[2] No one had exactly the same activity level score across all waves of the study, so no stability category was needed.

deviations. The 15 percent of respondents who reported very sharp declines accounted for most of the decline from 1975 to 1995 in mean activity level scores for the 1995 respondents. Note that our operational definition of *increase* or *decline* was specific to each individual because it was anchored at their baseline activity level. In general, the respondents were active and remained so throughout the study, although sometimes at a slightly reduced overall level (25% of respondents fell into the category of just greater than 1 standard deviation decline in overall activity level).

Regression analysis provides another way to examine the long-term consistency of activity levels from 1975 to 1995. Baseline factors that could reasonably be expected to influence activity included age, gender, education, self-confidence, and goal directedness. The expectation was that being younger, male, and having higher education, self-confidence, and goal directedness in 1975 would be related positively to 1995 activity level. In addition, we hypothesized that 1995 self-rated health and functional capability would be related positively to 1995 activity level, based on the idea that health and functional capability are prerequisites for activity.

Table 3.6 shows the results of this regression analysis. Baseline measures of enabling psychological factors such as self-confidence or having many important personal goals had no influence on 1995 activity level, nor did sociodemographic factors of gender and education. Surprisingly, neither 1995 self-rated health nor 1995 functional capability was a significant predictor of 1995 activity level when age was controlled. Continuity in activity level from 1975 to 1995 accounted for the greatest amount of variation in 1995 activity level (beta = .541). Age was the other significant factor (beta =

TABLE 3.6. Predictors of 1995 activity level ($N = 184$)

Predictor	Standardized Regression Coefficient
Age	−.225*
Education	.034
Gender	.008
1975	
Self-confidence	.026
Goal directedness	.067
Activity level	.541*
1995	
Self-rated health	.094
Functional capability	.067
Adjusted R^2	.356

* Beta coefficient significant at the .01 level or better.

$-.225$), and as expected, younger age predicted higher activity level. The adjusted R^2 for this model is .356, a modest result. This means that if we knew the respondent's 1975 activity level and age, controlling for the effects of other independent variables, these two variables would allow us to reduce error in predicting the respondent's 1995 activity level by 35.6 percent over predictions made at random or by chance. Of these two effective predictors, continuity in activity level was by far the most powerful.

To learn more about individual patterns within activity categories, we performed a series of analyses that looked at individual patterns of stability, continuity, and discontinuity within eight activity categories: being with friends, being with children and grandchildren, gardening, attending church functions, participating in civic organizations, doing handiwork, collecting, and reading. As mentioned, these categories are representative of the more abstract categories we identified through factor analysis.

Tracing individual activity patterns is a complex task. To be selected for this analysis, 1995 respondents had to have responded to at least three of the six survey waves, including the final two waves (the latter requirement was designed to provide a final baseline). *Stability* for each activity was defined as having the same item score for all survey waves. However, stability could occur at any of six levels of participation, ranging from "very often" (6) to "never" (1). *Continuity* was defined as fluctuations of no more than 1 item scale point. For example, a pattern of 6-5-5-6-6-5 would be classified as continuity in the "often" category because all responses were in the "often" or "very often" category. The "often" category of continuity could also include a pattern of 5-4-5-4-5-5 because most of the responses were "often." A pattern of 4-4-4-3-3-4 was classified as continuity in the "occasional" category because all responses were either "sometimes" or "seldom." Likewise, a pattern of 2-3-3-2-3-3 would also be classified as continuity in the "occasional" category (all responses were "seldom" or "very seldom"). A pattern of 2-1-1-1-2-1 was classified as continuity based in the "never" category because most of the responses, including the final one, were "never." Taking differences in the beginning level of participation into account, there were more than 25 possible patterns of continuity.

Discontinuity was defined operationally as a fluctuation of 2 or more item scale points. There were more than 30 patterns of discontinuity, but again the basic patterns of participation over time were: decreasing participation, increasing participation, U-shaped pattern, inverted U-shaped pattern, and other. Discontinuity could occur from several beginning points. For example, patterns of decline included such diverse combinations as 6-6-4-4-2-2,

6-6-6-4-4-4, and 4-3-1-1-1-1. Increases could range from 1-1-4-5-6-6 to 4-4-4-6-6-6. Examples of U-shaped patterns are 6-5-4-4-5-6, 3-3-1-1-2-3, and 5-3-3-3-5-5. An inverted U-shaped pattern could be 1-1-4-4-1-1, 4-4-6-6-4-4, or 2-3-4-4-2-2. Discontinuity patterns in the "other" category included W patterns (4-2-4-4-2-5), M patterns (1-4-1-4-1-1), N patterns (1-1-4-1-4-4), and backward N patterns (6-6-4-6-6-4). Note that the U-shaped, W-shaped, and N-shaped patterns all involved increases at the end of the pattern, and the inverted U, M, and backward N all involved declines at the end. But because of the frequent up-and-down nature of patterns in the "other" category, we are less confident that the last intervals represent a trend of increase or decrease compared with patterns that increased or decreased steadily over the course of the study. Some patterns in the "other" category could not be be assigned easily to a subcategory (e.g., 2-6-4-5-1-2).

Table 3.7 shows the data for all eight activities I consider in detail, classified by type of pattern. For convenience, I collapsed the data on frequency of participation from six categories to three: "often" ("often" or "very often"), "occasionally" ("sometimes," "seldom," and "very seldom"), and "never." I consider in turn patterns of stability, continuity, discontinuity, and stability and continuity combined.

For the eight activities shown in Table 3.7, stability is not common, and one of the greatest proportions of stability was produced by the 15.6 percent of respondents who *never* engaged in collecting. But for most activities, the "often" category was the most common form of stability in participation. Reading was the most common activity showing stability in the "often" category (24.3%).

Continuity of participation also largely occurred in the "often" category, especially for being with friends, being with children and grandchildren, gardening, and reading. But for attending church functions and handiwork, the proportion in the "often" category was not very different from the proportion in the "occasionally" category. Continuity of occasional participation was the norm for community organizations, and "never" was the most common form of continuity for collecting.

Discontinuity also varied considerably by type of activity. Increases in activity were most common for participation in civic organizations (16.2%) and attending church functions (10.1%). Most increases represented a movement from "occasionally" to "often."

Decreases were most common for gardening (27.5%), and most of these decreases were from "often" to "occasionally." Gardening usually involves the physical capability to grasp, lift, carry, and bend. Slightly greater than 23

TABLE 3.7. Patterns of activity, by activity type, 1975 to 1995 ($N = 309$)

	Children and Grandchildren	Friends	Gardening	Attending Church	Civic Organizations	Handiwork	Collecting	Reading
Stable	15.2%	16.6%	8.4%	15.4%	9.1%	9.4%	19.8%	25.6%
Often	9.1	10.4	5.8	8.5	1.0	4.2	2.6	24.3
Occasionally	3.2	6.2	2.6	1.6	1.9	1.6	1.6	1.3
Never	2.9			5.3	6.2	3.6	15.6	
Continuity	52.3	58.8	48.2	51.5	34.7	38.6	38.3	57.9
Often	32.7	34.8	29.8	22.3	10.1	14.9	3.6	48.2
Occasionally	15.9	23.7	16.8	19.1	16.9	15.3	14.6	9.7
Never	3.6	0.3	1.6	10.1	7.7	8.4	20.1	
Discontinuity	30.2	23.3	42.7	32.8	56.1	49.7	39.6	15.2
Increase	5.5	3.2	5.5	10.1	16.2	5.2	3.9	6.1
to "often"	5.2	2.6	4.9	8.5	9.7	1.6	0.6	5.5
to "occasionally"	0.3	0.6	0.6	1.6	6.5	3.6	3.3	0.6
Decrease	14.3	12.6	27.5	13.1	17.8	23.4	20.8	3.9
to "occasionally"	10.1	12.3	16.2	7.2	8.1	13.7	7.8	2.0
to "never"	4.2	0.3	11.3	5.9	9.7	9.7	13.0	1.9
U	4.9	4.6	6.9	3.6	9.1	5.2	5.5	2.6
to "often"	3.3	3.3	3.9	1.3	4.2	1.6	2.6	1.6
to "occasionally"	1.6	1.3	3.0	2.3	4.9	3.6	2.9	1.0
∩	2.6	0.6	1.9	4.5	8.4	8.4	3.6	1.3
to "occasionally"	2.3	0.6	1.9	4.2	5.2	2.9	0.6	1.3
to "never"	0.3			0.3	3.2	5.5	3.0	
Other	2.9	2.3	0.9	1.3	4.5	7.5	5.8	1.3
Omitted	2.3	1.3	0.6	0.3	0.3	2.3	2.3	1.3
Stable + Continuity	67.5	75.4	56.6	66.9	43.8	48.0	58.1	83.5
Often	41.8	45.2	35.6	30.8	11.1	19.1	6.2	72.5
Occasionally	19.2	29.9	19.4	20.7	18.8	16.9	16.2	11.0
Never	6.5	0.3	1.6	15.4	13.9	12.0	35.7	

percent of respondents reported a decrease in the frequency they engaged in handiwork; 13.7 percent moved from the "often" category to the "occasionally" category, but 9.7 percent dropped handiwork completely. For men, the handiwork category included woodworking and metalworking, which also involve physical capability. For women, handiwork was more likely to involve knitting, crocheting, or sewing, which also involve an element of physical capability but probably less than that comprising men's handiwork. Of the 20.8 percent who reported decreased participation in collecting, 7.8 percent had dropped from "often" to "occasionally," and 13 percent had dropped the activity completely. Of the 17.8 percent who declined in participation in civic organizations, 8.1 percent became "occasional" participants, and 9.7 percent dropped the activity entirely.

Thus, a relatively small proportion of the panel experienced activity losses in the absolute sense of dropping an activity in which they had participated at an earlier time. The more common pattern was to cut back participation to a lower level and retain the activity within the person's concept of his or her lifestyle. I will return to this theme later when I look at specific case examples.

U-shaped patterns of discontinuity were uncommon, but they occurred most frequently in participation in civic organizations (9.1% showed U-shaped patterns, and 8.4% showed inverted U-shaped patterns). Of the 50 respondents who increased their participation in civic organizations from "never" to "occasionally" or "often" during the study, 19 subsequently dropped out (inverted U). Of the 28 respondents with a U-shaped pattern of participation in civic organizations, 13 of them went from "often" to "occasionally" and then back to "often," and 15 went from "occasionally" to "never" back to "occasionally."

Taking up activities one had not done before was very uncommon in the the OLSAA. Even increases in activity occur within the context of a continuing array of activities. Participating in civic organizations showed a significant proportion of respondents (16.2%) moving from "never" having done the activity (at least during our study) to some level of participation. Handiwork was the other activity that showed a perceptible proportion taking up the activity from having "never" having done it earlier; ten respondents took up handiwork, but six of them eventually dropped it.

Participation in senior citizens organizations, not included in the original activity scale but added to the study in 1979, was another activity that increased significantly over time as the younger study respondents passed age 65. For example, among 162 respondents who were in their late 50s in 1979 (mean age 58.2), only 3 (1.5%) reported participating "often" or "very often" in senior citizens organizations. But by 1995, when this age cohort had an average age of 74.1, the number participating in senior citizens organizations "often" or "very often" had increased to 26 (16%). In the overall 1995 panel of respondents, 185 (74%) had reported "never" participating in senior citizens organizations in 1979, but that number had dropped to 73 (29.1%) by 1995. About 42 percent of the panel experienced discontinuity in relation to participation in senior citizens organizations, and nearly all of this discontinuity consisted of significantly increased participation. This stands to reason. Senior citizens organizations have a minimum age of eligibility (usually 60), and the median age of senior center participants is older than 75. This means that many panel respondents were below the eligibility age or the normative age for participation until much later in the study.

We also did not include household work or resting in our baseline activity inventory, but we did include them beginning in 1991. A very high proportion of respondents reported doing household work "often" or "very often" (87.2% in 1991 and 80.3% in 1995). The drop from 1991 to 1995 was statistically significant at the .05 level, therefore we can treat this as a real change and not just a random fluctuation. In 1991 not quite one third (32.6%) of respondents reported resting "often" or "very often," and this proportion increased to 45.5 percent by 1995, again a significant difference. However, the proportion that showed discontinuity in household work or resting between 1991 and 1995 was small (10% for household work and 11.9% for resting).

Table 3.7 also shows the combined data for both stability and continuity because stability is a form of continuity. A strong majority of respondents reported continuity in their patterns of activity participation in reading (83.5%) and being with friends (75.4%). A two-thirds majority reported continuity in being with children and grandchildren (67.5%) and attending church functions (66.9%), and a bare majority reported continuity in gardening (56.6%) and collecting (58.1%). However, the data for collecting are a bit misleading because most of the continuity in collecting comes from those who never participated. For the other activities, participating often is the most common form of continuity.

With all of the comings and goings in participation in civic organizations, it is not surprising that this activity did not show a majority of continuity patterns (it stands at 43% continuity). Likewise, many respondents engaged in handiwork episodically, so it is unsurprising that this activity shows less than a majority with continuity (48%).

Overall, continuity of activities was the norm for the OLSAA respondents over the 20 years of the study. Most respondents continued to engage in their customary activities at a consistent level over the entire period of the study. Those whose activity participation increased most often increased their participation level for activities they had been doing all along. Very few respondents took up new types of activities during the study, and joining civic organizations was by far the most common new activity. But many of those who took up new activities soon tired of them and tended to drop or cut back their participation. Respondents whose activity levels decreased tended to retain their involvement in the activity but at a reduced level. Very few respondents dropped activities. Gardening and handiwork were usually dropped for physical reasons, whereas the motivation for dropping collecting and civic organization participation had more to do with a diminished interest in these activities. Many respondents became bored with civic organizations and adopted a "been there, done that" attitude. Collectors tended to retain their collections of coins, antiques, rocks, or whatever, but they simply stopped acquiring new items.

In the longitudinal records, we see high and consistent participation in activities that involve socializing with others. In terms of organizational participation, attending church functions was much more likely to show a continuity pattern (66.9%) compared with participating in civic organizations (43.8%). Because gardening usually requires the ability to grasp, lift, carry, and bend, it is very vulnerable to impairments such as arthritis or diseases of the bones or joints. As a result, gardening sometimes had to be given up (11.3%). Nevertheless, most respondents showed a consistent pattern of gardening (56.6%), and very few had never gardened. Hobbies such as handiwork or collecting showed 48 and 58.1 percent continuity, respectively, over the course of the study, but part of this consistency occurred among people who never engaged in these activities at any point in the study. Hobbies showed the largest percentage of respondents with complex, up-and-down patterns such as the U, inverted U, W, M, or N, which means that their participation tended to be episodic. For example, 21.1 percent of the respondents reported one of the fluctuating patterns of discontinuity in their involvement with handiwork, and 14.9 percent showed fluctuating discontinuity in collecting. These proportions are relatively high compared with the proportions reporting fluctuating discontinuity for such activities as being with friends (7.5%) or attending church functions (9.4%). Finally, reading is a solitary activity that is very much under the control of each individual, and reading shows the highest level of consistency over the study (83.5%); a very large proportion (72.5%) reported reading often throughout the study. Only 1.9 percent reported that they never engaged in reading.

These data show that overall activity levels are a combination of separate activities with very different longitudinal profiles. In the next section, I look at activity patterns in a more holistic fashion.

How Activities Fit Together to Form Lifestyles

Earlier in this chapter, I discussed how activities could be classified into broad categories of emphasis: socializing, physical activity, organizational participation, hobbies, and solitary activities. We can use this same set of concepts to develop a view of how activities fit together to form lifestyles. Lifestyles can be *focused*, dominated by one of the broad categories listed above. In addition, lifestyles can incorporate frequent participation in all of the broad activity categories, in which case we could call the lifestyle *diversified*. On the other hand, lifestyles can reflect *minimal involvement* in any of the activity categories. In this section, I provide case illustrations of external continuity from each of these lifestyle categories.

Diversified

Kay had one of the highest activity levels throughout the study, more than 2 standard deviations above the mean for each survey wave. She was a never-employed homemaker who remained married throughout our study. She rated her health as very good throughout. Kay was heavily involved in all of our broad activity categories. She socialized very often with family and friends, played cards with friends, and attended social gatherings; she also participated in sports, gardening, and travel very often, all involving physical activity. She engaged in hobbies such as handiwork and in solitary activities such as participatory art and reading very often, and she participated in activities of community organizations and her church.

Kay's high degree of continuity in overall activity level was achieved through some trade-offs. For example, early in our study, when she was in her late 50s and early 60s, her physical activities included playing tennis and golf. But by age 63 she began to cut back on sports, and by age 77 she never participated in these activities. She offset this decline by increasing her involvement with gardening and travel. She also reduced her involvement in political organizations and offset the decline with increased participation in community service organizations.

Some keys to Kay's capacity to maintain very high activity levels and a diversified lifestyle included an extremely happy marriage that remained intact throughout the study, a college education, adequate income, very good health, continued residence in a familiar community and in the same dwelling, and children and grandchildren who continued to live nearby.

Socializing

The activities revolving around socializing included visiting with friends and family, attending social functions, and playing cards or board games. In addition, attending sporting events and travel were often forms of socializing. Spectator art such as attending concerts or visiting museums was also a form of socializing for women, and participatory sports often had an element of socializing for men.

Aside from reading and watching television, the only activities Cathy engaged in often or very often over the entire course of the study were attending social gatherings, visiting with friends, traveling, and playing cards. She very seldom or never participated in any form of organization, including church. She sometimes reported occasional participation in art, handiwork, or collecting but had no sustained participation. Her overall activity level was average and very consistent over the six waves of the study. Cathy was 86 in 1995. She had never married, and she had no children or grandchildren. She reported good health and adequate income throughout the study.

Stephen showed a similar pattern of having few activities that did not involve socializing. Aside from reading and watching television, the only activities that he engaged in often or very often over the course of the study were visiting with friends and family, attending social gatherings, traveling, attending sporting events, playing cards, and playing golf with his friends. He rarely participated in most of the other activity categories, including gardening, hobbies, or organizational involvement. His overall activity level was about average and was very consistent over the six waves of the study. At age 81 in 1995, Stephen was happily married and reported very good health and adequate income throughout the study.

Physical Activity

Ken devoted most of his discretionary time to physical activities — yardwork, hiking, cycling, and playing golf. He often spent time with family and friends, and he read a lot, but his passion was exercising his body. Unlike the cases above, where participating in sports was used as a vehicle for socializing, Ken usually performed these activities alone. Except for attending church functions frequently, Ken was very uninvolved in formal organizations in the community. His lifestyle revolved around physical activity, but he also had a strong marriage that provided emotional support. At age 73 in 1995, Ken was one of the younger members of the panel. He was a highly educated retired executive who reported very good health and income adequacy throughout the study.

Organizational Participation

Dorothy's lifestyle focused on formal organizations in the community. A shy widow, Dorothy was a member of more than a dozen groups, including those in her church, several community service organizations, those concerned with social justice, and three music groups. She had very little free time for hobbies or solitary pursuits other than reading. Her socializing took place within the context of her group participation, and she linked her identity very solidly to being a steady and responsible group participant. She seldom just got together with friends, and she had no family living in the community. Her only physical activity was taking care of her yard, which for her was a task that needed doing rather than a satisfying activity.

Hobbies

Lyle's lifestyle revolved around exercising his skills in manual arts. Although he had spent his occupational career as a college professor, Lyle was an expert furniture maker and carpenter. He also restored antique furniture and supervised construction for a local Habitat for Humanity organization. Handiwork was the only activity that Lyle reported doing very often throughout the course of the study, and he was involved only in organizations that used his carpentry knowledge. He was very committed to helping the disadvantaged, and he donated the proceeds from his handiwork to local charities. Lyle reported that he read or watched television only occasionally, and he found plenty of physical exercise in his furniture and home building. Lyle was a quiet man with little need for socializing or organizational involvement. He preferred to spend his time quietly working alone. Nevertheless, he was happily married throughout the study, and he reported consistently very good health and adequate income.

Solitary Activities

John's lifestyle stressed solitary activities. Although he was happily married throughout the study, John spent most of his free time alone reading, doing woodworking projects, tending his coin collection, or working on his extensive model railroad. He never participated in any form of organization. He had few friends and visited with them only occasionally. His main form of socializing was visiting with his children and grandchildren. John's activity level was below average for the panel throughout the study, but his array of activities was very consistent. He was in good health and had adequate income throughout the study.

Minimal Involvement

Minimal involvement is the opposite of the diversified activity pattern: the diversified lifestyle involves frequent participation in a large array of activities, but minimal involvement means seldom or never participating in them. People with this lifestyle tend to be lifelong loners.

> Throughout the entire study, the only activity that Patrick reported doing often was listening to the news and music on public radio. Patrick never married, had no family living in the community, and lived alone throughout the study in the home he had occupied with his parents, who had died many years before our study began. He spent his days doing work around the house and in the yard, and he derived satisfaction from being able to remain self-reliant. He was almost completely separated from the world of leisure activities that framed the lifestyles of his neighbors in the community. His energies were occupied by an internal world of keeping up with current events on the radio and enjoying nature. He had no organizational involvements and a few acquaintances but no ongoing friendships. He had no hobbies and was a lifelong isolate whose home environment had for many years shown the pattern of clutter and shabbiness that conforms to the stereotype of the elderly hermit.
>
> Although he reported being lonely a lot, Patrick was generally very happy with his situation. His morale was average, and his attitude toward his life in retirement was among the most positive in the panel. Although his overall activity level was far below average throughout the study, and his pattern of nontraditional activity was very consistent, Patrick was very satisfied with how he spent his time.
>
> Patrick was in his early 80s in 1995. He was in good health throughout the study, and he reported that his income improved from inadequate to adequate after 1979, when he was able to draw Social Security retirement benefits.

These case histories indicate that activity patterns are highly individualized but can be classified into broad categories. Of the respondents showing a pattern of continuity in activities over the course of the study, 55 percent showed a diversified activity pattern. This is not surprising given the generally high activity levels in the panel. A lifestyle focused on socializing accounted for 25 percent of those showing continuity in lifestyle; lifestyles focused on hobbies or organizational participation accounted for 7 percent each. Lifestyles focused on physical activity or solitary activities made up just under 6 percent combined, and minimal involvement accounted for less than 1 percent.

Note that in most of the cases cited, good health and adequate income played important supporting roles in maintaining continuity of activity patterns over time. Note also that in several cases continuity of lifestyle patterns was achieved by offsetting increases and decreases in specific activities within general activity categories. Thus, once again we see that continuity means preserving a general pattern and that specific change can often be accommodated within such general patterns.

Summary

In this chapter I have looked at external continuity from a number of perspectives: continuity of dwelling, household composition, and community; continuity of activity patterns measured in several different ways; and continuity of lifestyles. External continuity is very prevalent in our panel, especially for income adequacy, dwelling, household composition, and community of residence. Only 14 percent of our 1995 respondents experienced a change in both household composition and residence. Only 15 percent reported that their income was inadequate at any time during the study. Only 16 percent were dependent on others for transportation at any time in the study. Thus, in terms of the basic structural elements of lifestyle, continuity was by far the most common experience. Even when I looked at complex patterns of activities over time, I found that continuity was the most common outcome.

However, external continuity was not simply the result of inertia or habit. The respondents' levels of activity were most definitely influenced by their prior activity levels. In lagged regression analyses, prior activity level was the strongest predictor of current activity level; however, age negatively influenced activity level in some of the analyses, and current self-confidence was also a significant predictor of activity level in the early stages of the survey. In combination, these factors accounted for a large proportion (around 66%) of the variation in activity level. This is a high degree of association for survey research involving social and social psychological variables.

I also found that continuity in overall activity levels was often achieved by offsetting increases and decreases in specific activity types. As the age of the panel increased, the mean activity level dropped. In this context, it is important that more than 50 percent of the panel showed continuity in their activity levels. The drop in mean overall activity level was accounted for mostly by the 15 percent of respondents who reported very sharp declines in overall activity level.

When I looked at the sources of continuity in activity patterns, I found that more than two thirds of the panel reported continuity in reading, visiting with friends, visiting with children and grandchildren, and attending church functions. Note that continuity need not imply frequent participation, but for the activities just mentioned, the most common pattern was frequent participation.

Overall, continuity of activities was the norm for panel respondents over the 20-year course of the study. Most respondents continued to engage in their customary activities at their customary level of participation. Those who became more active tended to increase their participation in activities they had been doing all along. Very few took up new types of activity during the study. Those who reduced their overall activity level tended to maintain their array of activity but at a lower level of participation.

I also looked at the extent to which activity profiles could be organized into identifiable lifestyles and found that the general activity types lent themselves very well to this type of analysis. I presented examples of specific lifestyles that fit the various types. Of the majority of respondents who fit into a continuity pattern of activities, 55 percent had a diversified lifestyle pattern in which they participated often in at least one activity in each of the general activity areas: socializing, hobbies, organizational participation, physical activity, and solitary pursuits. Another 25 percent of respondents had lifestyles that revolved around socializing. Hobbies, organizational participation, physical activity, and solitary activities were the core of lifestyles for a relatively small proportion of respondents. Minimal involvement, which was a lifestyle that did not involve more than very occasional participation in the types of activity that made up our activity types, was rare. But for those who chose a lifelong isolated and solitary lifestyle, the result was not necessarily negative in terms of morale or appreciation of life.

4 | Adaptive Capacity

What about aging requires adaptation? Many physical, psychological, and social changes that accompany aging alter individuals' circumstances in ways that require people to make some sort of adjustment. Sometimes people must adapt to positive changes such as moving to a healthier environment or getting accustomed to more freedom and autonomy after retirement. The processes of physical aging can result in physical constraints that require compensation and adaptation. Aging sometimes brings increasing financial constraints that require lifestyle modifications. Both physical and financial limitations can alter the capacity to preserve an individual's preferred lifestyle. Aging can also alter relationships, as friends and family members themselves face physical and financial limitations associated with aging or as cherished friends and relatives move to another community or die. All of these changes require some form of adaptation.

Adaptation is the process of adjusting to fit a situation or environment. It is actually several processes that individuals use to deal with constant changes encountered in daily living. Changes that require adaptation can occur in ourselves, in our situations, or in our environments. Early in adulthood, most of us develop routine strategies for dealing with change. Each of us can adjust to a certain amount of change nearly automatically, without special effort and sometimes without even being aware of having adapted. However, some changes surpass our capacity for routine adaptation and require that we take unusual, nonroutine steps to deal with them.

Coping means contending with or attempting to overcome difficulty. Over time, we develop coping strategies and skills that we use to grapple with significant changes in circumstances. Coping strategies may evolve over time as we learn more about how to use them, but it is common for people to use consistent coping strategies throughout adulthood, as continuity theory predicts.

People adapt to aging in two major ways: by gradual, routine adaptation and by mobilizing coping skills and resources to deal with crises. Many age changes occur gradually and can be accommodated routinely (Pearlin 1991). Other changes may be accommodated routinely at first, but eventually they may accumulate to a point that exceeds a person's threshold for routine adaptation and requires major adjustments and a corresponding mobilization of personal and social resources. Still other changes may be both sudden and serious and require immediate conscious coping and social support (Pearlin 1991). For example, people usually adapt to age changes in appearance gradually and routinely. Adaptation to increasing physical frailty may be gradual at first, but when individuals begin to lose needed functional capabilities, adaptation requires more conscious planning and decision making and more social support. Changes that are sudden and profound, such as serious paralyzing strokes or disabilities resulting from serious accidents, are the greatest coping challenge for most people. Compared with the difficulties involved in coping with the effects of sudden and profound disability, adaptation to the usual pattern of gradual physical aging or to social role changes in later life, such as retirement or widowhood, is much easier and much more amenable to continuity solutions.

From a phenomenological or personal construct perspective (Ryff 1984; Kelly 1955), coping involves using psychological processes to ameliorate or neutralize potential negative effects of stress that might be associated with having to adapt. Pearlin (1991, 330) suggested that adults have "a large inventory of perceptual and cognitive devices" that enable them to view their problems as relatively minor. Through these devices, adults define situations or problems in ways that lessen perceptions of threat and, as a result, lessen stressful impact. Pearlin felt that although perceptual or cognitive coping does not eliminate the problem, such coping does control and shape the meaning of the situation or problem in a positive way, and potentially "stressful effects are buffered." Pearlin also felt that selective use of "socially valued goals and activities" is an important part of perceptual and cognitive coping. Thus, internal and external continuity both represent resources that are used in coping. This perspective helps us understand why transitions such as retirement are seldom experienced as stressful, even though scholars have often expected them to be (Skaff 1995).

Adaptive capacity is the core of adult development, according to continuity theory. By middle age, most adults have firm ideas about what their adaptive strengths and weaknesses are. They use these ideas to make choices that they see as leading to their strengths and minimizing their weaknesses. As they continue to evolve, adults also have increasingly firm ideas about what gives them satisfaction in life, and maintaining links to those sources of satisfaction is an important strategy for adapting to change. Internal and external continuity are outcomes of past choices, but a desire to maintain continuity can also be the foundation for future choices as well.

Adaptive capacity is the extent to which an individual has the social resources and orientations needed to adapt to significant changes in physical and social circumstances. Having the capacity to adapt means being able to make sense out of changes and to make effective decisions in response to them. Adaptive capacity is also involved in coping with internal or external changes that individuals themselves initiate as part of their goals for developmental direction.

Adaptation is made much easier by continuity in basic coping resources such as adequate income, good health, high physical functioning, and adequate social support. When losses occur in these basic coping resources, individuals can compensate by relying more on those that remain. But we would expect that people who experience losses in all resources for adaptation would have much greater difficulty adapting to change compared with people whose basic coping resources remain intact.

In addition to basic coping resources, adaptation is enhanced by mental orientations that reflect a sense of self-efficacy or agency, provide guidance for making decisions, prevent losses in basic coping resources, and point to customary strategies for adaptation. According to continuity theory, individuals actively construct their perceptions of problems, solutions, and outcomes. But they also interpret their experiences and use this feedback from experience to refine their ideas about how best to adapt to significant change.

In this chapter, I look first at coping resources people use to adapt and how coping strategies relate to motivation for continuity. Then I consider continuity in basic coping resources followed by a consideration of how people fare in coping with substantial changes in circumstances brought on by retirement, widowhood, and loss of functional capability.

Proactive Coping and Motivation for Continuity

Many people attempt to influence the pathways that their internal and external lives take. They make plans, and they use their values and beliefs to anticipate future needs. Years ago I hypothesized that expected life events such as retirement did not produce life crises because people can anticipate and plan for these transitions (Atchley 1975b). We could call this process

TABLE 4.1. Multidimensional scale of Orientation toward Continuity (*N* = 264)

Item	Agree (%)	Disagree (%)
Often, I do not really make decisions; I just let things happen.		78.6
When I need to solve problems, I usually try solutions that have worked for me before.	91.9	
I know myself well enough to know which choices are best for me.	96.3	
Over the years, I have continued activities that suit me and discontinued ones that do not.	96.3	
My choices seldom turn out as well as I expect.		87.5
I have no sense of the direction I want my life to take.		91.5
My philosophy of life is a consistent force behind the decisions I make.	88.6	
My basic lifestyle has changed significantly in the past ten years.		55.5
Most of my friends are people I first met within the past ten years.		73.7
My basic beliefs and values have changed significantly in the past ten years.		86.7

proactive coping. People cope by anticipating problems and creating conditions that neutralize potential difficulties that might arise.

Perhaps the most important question for this book is whether people see themselves as using continuity as a proactive adaptive strategy. To get at this question, we developed a ten-item scale we call Orientation toward Continuity. The items and the percentage of 1995 respondents who endorsed a positive value related to disposition toward continuity for each item are shown in Table 4.1. This scale is distributed normally within the positive conceptual space of disposition toward continuity, with a range of 21 to 40, a mean of 30.1, and a standard deviation of 3.1. None of the respondents had a score that reflected a disposition away from continuity. Some might think that this reflects a defect in the scale, that some people must have no interest in continuity; but continuity theory leads us to expect such people to be extremely rare. To want a preponderance of discontinuity would be to want no firm basis for psychological or social security, and most people do not desire such a state.

The respondents overwhelmingly endorsed the tenets of continuity theory. They make conscious decisions rather than just letting things happen (78.6% agreed), and they do experience predictable results from their choices (87% disagreed that their choices seldom turn out as expected). They usually try solutions that have worked for them in the past (91.9% agreed), they know themselves well enough to make choices that fit for them (96.3%

agreed), and they have indeed continued activities that suit them and discontinued those that do not (96.3% agreed). They have a sense of the developmental direction they want their life to take (91.5% disagreed that they had no such sense of direction), and they have a philosophy of life that provides a consistent force behind their decisions (88.6% agreed).

In terms of their subjective perceptions of internal and external continuity, a majority (55.5%) disagreed with the statement that their lifestyle has changed significantly, 73.7 percent disagreed that they met most of their friends in the last ten years (most of their friendships were longstanding), and 86.7 percent did not believe that their basic beliefs and values had changed significantly over the past decade. These subjective perceptions of continuity coincide very well with the objective measures of internal and external continuity presented in Chapters 2 and 3.

Thus, respondents overwhelmingly see themselves as using continuity as an adaptive coping strategy and as having a high degree of internal and external continuity. Some might contend that these findings are not evidence of active continuity but instead are simply the result of behavioral rigidity. To test this idea, we looked at the correlation between scores on a 14-item subset of the Wesley Mental Rigidity Inventory (Wesley 1953) and scores on our scale of disposition toward continuity. The scales were not significantly correlated (Pearson correlation = .038). Wesley's rigidity scale measures the extent to which people have set and methodical ways of dealing with the details of life, whereas the disposition toward continuity scale measures more general orientations. Some people who were high in disposition toward continuity were also high in rigidity, but an equal number were not. I now turn to other evidence that respondents attempt to create continuity proactively.

TABLE 4.2. Multidimensional scale of preventive health practices (N = 309)

Over the past 20 years, how often have you performed the following activities?

Activity	Frequency (%)[a]				
	Always	Usually	Sometimes	Seldom	Never
Complete physical exam at least every three years	43.0	25.9	10.4	13.3	6.1
Ate a balanced, fat-restricted diet	20.4	55.3	17.5	4.2	1.6
Attempted to maintain a desired weight	34.0	44.3	11.7	5.2	2.9
Used car seatbelts	77.7	14.2	5.2	1.6	0.3
Participated in physical exercise	37.5	31.4	20.4	7.1	2.6
Limited alcohol consumption	62.8	24.6	6.1	1.9	3.6
Avoided use of tobacco	82.2	4.2	1.0	2.9	8.4
Followed directions for taking prescription medications	85.1	12.0			0.6

[a] Rows do not add to 100 percent because of missing cases.

TABLE 4.3. Predictors of health variables, 1995

	Dependent Variable	
Predictor	1995 Self-Rated Health	1995 Functional Capability
Education	.094	.041
Gender	.051	.166**
1975 Activity level	.038	.075
Age	−.030	−.274**
1975 Functional capability		.218**
1975 Self-rated health	.590**	
Preventive health practices	.112*	.211**
Adjusted R^2	.360	.240
N	252	250

* Beta coefficient significant at the .05 level or better.
** Beta coefficient significant at the .001 level or better.

Not only did respondents attempt to create continuity in their lifestyles and relationships, they also tried to produce continuity in health and functioning as well. We asked the respondents how often over the 20 years of the study they had engaged in a series of preventive health practices. The items and the distribution of 1995 responses are shown in Table 4.2. The results clearly indicate why the panel is generally in good health. A large majority has always or usually followed the conventional wisdom about how to promote good health. They had physical examinations at least every three years, watched their diets, attempted to control their weight, used car seat belts, exercised, limited their alcohol consumption, avoided tobacco, and followed the directions in using prescription drugs. And these preventive health measures paid off for the majority who used them.

Table 4.3 shows the results of a regression analysis predicting 1995 functional capability from baseline functional capability in 1975, age, gender, education, 1975 activity level, and preventive health practices. A high score on preventive health practices was indeed significantly related to high functional capability. In addition, high 1995 functional capability was also predicted by high baseline functional capability, being of a younger age, and being male. Education and 1975 activity level were not significant predictors of 1995 functional capability.

A second analysis predicted 1995 self-rated health using this same approach. In these results, only high baseline self-rated health and high preventive health practices predicted high 1995 self-rated health. None of the other independent variables, including gender, was a significant predictor. Again, these longitudinal results show that respondents who use preventive coping strategies got results; they had higher self-rated health than respondents who scored lower on preventive health practices.

How Did Respondents Cope?

We have seen that respondents proactively used continuity and preventive health strategies to produce positive life outcomes. But how did respondents cope with adversity? We asked the set of open-ended questions, "What enables you to cope? What keeps you going?" We coded up to five separate answers to this set of questions. Table 4.4 shows two levels of general categories of coping strategy that were developed from the responses to these items. Although the exact statements showed a high degree of individuation in their precise wording, the first-level general categories produced a high degree of inter-rater reliability in coding (98.7%).

We look at these responses in several ways: strategies reported by the 66 respondents who listed only one coping strategy, rankings of specific strategies across all 266 arrays, and the proportional ranking of each general coping strategy by order of mention.[1]

Among the 66 respondents (24.3% of the total) who listed only one coping strategy, a positive outlook ranked highest (22 cases), followed by religiousness (16 cases), and relationships (12 cases). Productive activity, situational resources, and strategies falling outside the classification scheme accounted for 5 cases each. One respondent reported having no choice but to cope but did not specify a strategy.

When we look at first-level strategies and the frequency with which they were mentioned, regardless of the order of mention, relationships occupy three of the top four rankings (family, 108 mentions; friends, 88 mentions; and marriage, 56 mentions). Religiousness ranked third with 79 mentions, a positive attitude had 53 mentions, keeping productively busy had 51, and good health had 46. All other specific strategies had fewer than 30 mentions.

Table 4.5 presents data on the proportion reporting both moderate- and higher-level categories of coping strategies. I focus the discussion on the most frequently mentioned higher-level categories (relationships, positive outlook, religiousness, productive activity, and situational factors). Again, relationships, positive outlooks, and religiousness stand out as the most often mentioned and first-mentioned coping strategies. Differences among the proportion of first mentions of these three are small. Situational factors and

[1] We compared self-rated health, activity level, and morale of the 43 respondents who did not respond to this question with those who did. The nonresponders had significantly lower morale but did not differ from responders in terms of activity level or self-rated health. One might hypothesize that the nonresponders had lower morale because they did not have identifiable coping strategies.

TABLE 4.4. Categories of coping strategies

What enables you to cope? What keeps you going?

Positive outlook

　Positive attitude: look at the bright side, cooperative, worry free, hope, happiness, love, sense of humor, belief in people, faith in people

　Perseverance: strong will, guts, determination, persistence, never give up

　Love of life: desire to live, lots of living to do, *joie de vivre*

　Self-concept: self-acceptance, self-esteem, good memories, values, able to be alone, enjoy little satisfactions

　Curiosity: keeping up with current events, how will things turn out?, desire to learn, desire for new experience

　Religiousness: faith, God's grace, prayer, spiritual journey, relationship with God

　Appreciation of nature: conservation, animals, birds, plants, garden

Relationships

　Marriage: husband, wife, positive relationship

　Family: children, grandchildren, great-grandchildren, siblings, etc.

　Friends: being with people, love of people, support from friends

Situational factors

　Good physical health

　Sound mind

　Comfortable situation: financial security, good place to live, safe, secure, satisfying lifestyle, comfortable routine, flexible schedule

Goals

　Productively busy (activities, interests): all types of leisure activities, employment, goals *except* service to others

　Service to others: being needed, volunteer work, making things better

　Responsibilities and obligations

Other

　No choice (respondent did not have a choice, had to get through it)

　Don't know

　Blank in an otherwise completed questionnaire

productive activities fall well behind the three leading strategies in terms of prevalence of mention.

　Given that religiousness consists of only one first-level category, whereas relationships and positive outlook are made up of three and five first-level categories each, religiousness is a prominent coping strategy for those respondents who choose it, but 70.3 percent of respondents who listed at least one coping strategy did not mention religiousness. Koenig (1994) reported that 24 percent of his community respondents age 70 or over spontaneously mentioned religion as a coping strategy, results not very different from the

TABLE 4.5. Frequency of mention for various coping strategies

	Order of Mention (%)				
	1	2	3	4	5
Relationships	23.5	31.0	16.5	7.2	3.2
Family	12.9	11.0	7.1	2.6	1.3
Friends	3.2	12.6	7.8	3.6	1.3
Marriage	7.4	7.4	1.6	1.0	0.6
Attitude	21.0	11.0	6.4	5.5	2.5
Positive attitude	7.4	3.2	3.9	1.9	0.6
Perseverance	3.2	1.9	0.3		
Love life	4.2	2.6	0.3	1.0	0.6
Self-concept	3.6	2.3	1.3	1.3	0.3
Curiosity	2.6	1.0	0.6	1.3	1.0
Religiousness	17.2	2.9	2.3	2.6	
Nature		0.3	1.0	0.6	1.3
Productive activity	5.7	8.7	6.8	5.1	2.0
Busy	4.5	3.9	3.9	3.2	1.0
Service	0.6	3.2	2.3	1.6	1.0
Responsibility	0.6	1.6	0.6	0.3	
Situation	10.0	6.5	5.1	2.0	3.2
Good health	8.1	2.3	1.9	1.0	1.6
Sound mind	0.3	1.6	0.3		
Comfortable situation	1.6	2.6	2.9	1.0	1.6
Other	13.9	2.3	3.6	1.3	0.6
No choice	0.6	0.3	0.3		
Don't know	2.3				
Blank	13.9	36.9	57.9	75.7	87.0

29.7 percent mentioning religious coping among our respondents, who were also age 70 or over when this question was asked in 1995.

When we look at first-mentioned coping strategies, men and women respondents tended to mention positive attitudes, relationships, and productive activities in about equal proportions. However, the proportion mentioning religiousness was significantly higher among women (25.1%) than among men (5.6%). On the other hand, men were more likely to omit this question (24.6%) compared with women (15.8%).

Second-mentioned coping strategies also showed important gender differences. Women (40.7%) were more likely to mention relationships than were men (24.6%); but men were more likely to mention using positive attitudes (15.1%) and productive activities (13.5%) compared with women (9.5% and 6.5%, respectively).

The strategies our respondents use to cope depend on maintaining internal continuity of positive outlooks and religiousness and external continuity of relationships and productive activities. A few of our respondents also depended on being able to count on continuing good physical and mental health and material resources. As we saw in Chapters 2 and 3, continuity in these factors is a reasonable expectation.

Coping with Specific Changes: Retirement, Widowhood, and Functional Limitations

We saw earlier that our respondents were motivated to use continuity as a general coping strategy and that specific coping strategies usually depended on maintaining a certain amount of both internal and external continuity. In this section I look at how changes widely thought to be significant — retirement, widowhood, and the onset of functional limitations — influence continuity and whether being able to maintain continuity eases the effects of these changes in terms of maintaining a sense of psychological well-being. For each of the changes I consider, I use quantitative techniques to look at how the change influenced continuity of morale and activity level. Then I examine the impact of each of these changes in the context of internal and external continuity for specific cases.

Retirement

To understand the impact of retirement, before-and-after comparisons are an important tool. For example, in the first analysis I look at morale before and after retirement for those who retired between waves of the study. But it is also important to include information on morale for those who continued to be employed because morale can fluctuate within both groups. I then use a similar strategy to examine the relationship between retirement and activity level.

To measure change in morale, morale was recoded into five categories that correspond roughly to a mean category and categories plus or minus 1 and 2 standard deviations from the mean. Because the mean morale scores were quite stable across waves of the Ohio Longitudinal Study of Aging and Adaptation (OLSAA), the same categories could be used for all waves. Simply by cross-tabulating time 1 (T_1) and time 2 (T_2) morale scores, we can easily identify the proportion of cases that remained in same category and those that increased or decreased. However, this analysis is complicated by the fact that relatively few respondents retired within any one of the two-year intervals from 1975 to 1981. To provide a sufficient number of retirements for analysis, the data were combined to show before-and-after results for those who retired between T_1 and T_2, where T_1 and T_2 could be 1975 to 1977,

1977 to 1979, or 1979 to 1981. This combining of data resulted in data for 47 men and 44 women who retired within any two-year interval.

To know the effect of retirement on morale, we also need to compare change in morale among those who retired with change in morale among those who remained employed over similar two-year intervals. Table 4.6 shows how the basic tables used to do the comparative analysis were constructed. The top panel of Table 4.6 shows the data for 309 reports from men who were employed at both time points in each of three two-year intervals. The diagonal consists of those whose morale scores did not change (45%);

TABLE 4.6. Morale over two waves of measurement for men employed at both times and for men who were employed full-time at time 1 and retired at time 2

Men Employed T$_1$ and T$_2$	Morale T$_2$				
	1	2	3	4	5
Morale T$_1$					
Moderate					
1	14	5	3	3	
2	8	4	6	8	2
3	1	6	15	14	9
4	3	3	23	54	37
Very high					
5		4	5	30	52

	N	%
Increased morale T$_1$ to T$_2$	87	28.1[a]
Unchanged morale T$_1$ to T$_2$	139	45.0
Decreased morale T$_1$ to T$_2$	83	26.9
Total	309	

Men employed T$_1$ and retired T$_2$	Morale T$_2$				
	1	2	3	4	5
Morale T$_1$					
Moderate					
1	1	1	1	2	
2		1			1
3		1	2	3	2
4	1		3	9	11
Very high					
5		1		2	5

	N	%
Increased morale T$_1$ to T$_2$	21	44.6
Unchanged morale T$_1$ to T$_2$	18	38.3
Decreased morale T$_1$ to T$_2$	8	17.1
Total	47	

[a] Percentage differences between still employed and retired are significant at the .05 level (chi-square).

TABLE 4.7. Morale over two-year intervals, by employment status and gender

| | Morale | | | | | | | |
| | Total | | Increased | | Unchanged | | Decreased | |
Employment Status	N	%	N	%	N	%	N	%
Employed T₁ and T₂								
Men	309	100.0	87	28.1	139	45.0	83	26.9
Women	154	100.0	48	31.2	61	39.6	45	29.2
Employed T₁ and retired T₂								
Men	47	100.0	21	44.6*	18	38.3	8	17.1
Women	44	100.0	15	34.1	17	38.6	12	27.3

* Difference between still-employed and retired men is significant at the .05 level.

those above the diagonal (28.1%) showed an increase in morale over a two-year interval; and those below the diagonal (26.9%) showed a decrease in morale.

The bottom panel of Table 4.6 shows data for men who retired during a two-year survey interval. Among these 47 men, 38.3 percent showed no change in morale, 44.6 percent showed an increase, and 17.1 percent showed a decrease. After retirement, morale stayed the same or increased for 82.9 percent, so retirement was associated with maintained or enhanced morale for a large majority of men who retired.

These results take on added significance when we compare still-employed men with just-retired men in terms of the proportion with increased morale. Among just-retired men, 44.6 percent showed increased morale, and 17.1 percent showed decreased morale compared with their preretirement morale score. But among still-employed men, 28.1 percent showed increased morale, and 26.9 percent showed decreased morale. These differences between just-retired and still-employed men are statistically significant at the .05 level using the chi-square test of expected frequencies. Thus, retirement resulted in significantly more men with increased morale and significantly fewer men with decreased morale compared with data for the still-employed men. These data also show that men adapted to retirement very well.

Table 4.7 shows data on morale by gender for those who were employed at both times and for those who retired during a two-year interval. For women, retirement did not have the same positive effects on morale that it had for men. Over two-year intervals, still-employed men and women had similar profiles of increase and decrease in morale, and just-retired women had patterns of increase and decrease in morale that were not significantly different from those of still-employed men and women. Similar results were obtained in an analysis of morale over the ten-year 1981 to 1991 interval. Thus, adapta-

TABLE 4.8. Activity level over two-year intervals, by employment status and gender

| | Activity Level | | | | | | | |
| | Total | | Increased | | Unchanged | | Decreased | |
Employment Status	N	%	N	%	N	%	N	%
Employed T_1 and T_2								
Men	316	100.0	50	15.8	179	56.7	78	27.5
Women	166	100.0	26	15.7	96	57.8	44	26.5
Employed T_1 and retired T_2								
Men	47	100.0	5	10.6	25	53.2	17	36.2
Women	46	100.0	14	30.4*	22	47.8	10	21.8

* Difference between retired women and men is significant, and the difference between still-employed and retired women is significant (chi-square, .05 level).

tion patterns as reflected by overall morale score were not affected by retirement for women, but retirement affected adaptation among men positively.

Note, however, that most changes in morale occurred at the top end of the range of morale scores (see Table 4.6), so it would be erroneous to conclude that those with relatively low morale scores had substantively low morale. Decreases in morale tended to be concentrated at the upper end of the scale, as were increases in morale.

The data for morale show that adaptation results in maintenance or improvement in morale for all groups over two-year intervals, and the proportion showing increased morale is notably higher for just-retired men. Thus, internal continuity of adaptation is high for most respondents regardless of employment/retirement status, but for men it seems to be enhanced further by retirement.

Now I consider the impact of retirement on overall activity levels. Table 4.8 shows data on activity levels and was constructed in the same manner as Table 4.7. These data show that stability in activity level is more common than stability in morale; a majority of still-employed men and women and just-retired men had unchanged activity levels over a two-year interval. Increased activity level was much less common than increased morale for all groups except just-retired women, who showed a proportion with increased activity level comparable to their proportion with increase in morale (30.4% compared with 34.1%). Indeed, just-retired women were significantly more likely than still-employed men and women and just-retired men to show an increase in activity level over a two-year interval. On the other hand, just-retired men were significantly more likely to show a decrease in activity level compared with still-employed men, and just-retired men were also much more likely (36.2%) than just-retired women (21.8%) to show a decline in activity level. Thus, compared with their still-employed counterparts, just-retired women were more likely to increase activity, and just-retired men were more likely to decrease activity. The gender differences in activity level change were large and statistically significant among the just-retired persons.

However, it is important to focus on the context of these differences. The proportion maintaining or increasing their activity level over a two-year interval was quite high for all subgroups, ranging from 63.8 percent for just-retired men to 72.5 percent for still-employed men, to 73.5 percent for still-employed women, to 78.2 percent for just-retired women. Thus, if maintaining or increasing customary activity levels is considered a measure of adaptation, all groups showed high proportions who had adapted. Given that retirement increased morale more for men than for women, we could hardly argue that the lower activity levels for just-retired men are maladaptive. Instead, what is more likely is that retirement frees both men and women to take part in activity at a level closer to their ideal.

Widowhood

Using a quantitative approach to assess the impact of widowhood on the OLSAA respondents is difficult because very few respondents became widowed during any single survey interval, especially among men. In the first analysis, I look at the impact of widowhood on morale and activity level in the same manner that we assessed the impact of retirement. Table 4.9 shows data on morale and activity level for women who remained married and for women who became widowed over various survey waves. We combined the data for the three two-year intervals, and we included data from the 1981 to 1991 interval because more women became widowed during this interval. Because the number of women who became widowed is very small — 18 for all three two-year intervals and 34 for the ten-year interval — proportional differences between widows and women who continued to be married have to be very large (more than 20 percentage points difference) to be statistically significant at the .05 level, using chi-square. None of the differences in Table 4.9 is this large, which means that there is about a 10 percent probability that even the large differences we observe between still-married and widowed women could have occurred by chance and not because widows are actually different from still-married women. With this caveat, some of the results deserve comment, if only to suggest avenues for future research.

The proportion who maintained unchanged morale was much lower among widows than among still-married women for both the combined two-

TABLE 4.9. Morale and activity-level changes for widowed and for still-married women over two-year survey intervals

	Morale					
	Increased		Unchanged		Decreased	
	N	%	N	%	N	%
Married T_1 and T_2 ($N = 481$)	147	30.6	206	42.9	128	26.6
Married T_1 to widowed T_2 ($N = 18$)	7	38.9	5	27.8	6	33.3
	Activity Level					
Married T_1 and T_2 ($N = 515$)	83	16.1	276	53.6	156	30.3
Married T_1 to widowed T_2 ($N = 18$)	3	16.7	9	50.0	6	33.3

year interval data (27.8% versus 42.9%) and the ten-year interval (32.1% for widows versus 48.1% for still-married women). However, change in morale was bidirectional among widows, with more widows showing an increase in morale after widowhood compared with still-married women. But the proportion showing a decrease in morale was also higher among widows than among still-married women. These findings suggest that for some women, widowhood represented a relief from caregiving and worrying about their spouse's health, which in turn increased their morale. For others widowhood produced the expected disproportional decline in morale. As with our earlier analyses, it is important to remember that declines in morale were concentrated in the positive end of the morale distribution. But, unlike the analysis for retirement, where few respondents showed an extreme drop in morale after retirement, 17.5 percent (seven) of the women who became widowed dropped from an above-average morale to the lowest category. However, even those in the lowest morale category had only relatively low morale, not substantively low morale; that is, their morale scores were at the low end of the positive concept space in the morale scale.

Only 12 men became widowed during the first six years of the OLSAA, not enough to do a quantitative analysis. However, 5 of the 12 (41.7%) suffered a substantial drop in morale compared with only 12.2 percent reporting a substantial drop among men who remained married over the two-year intervals.

Table 4.9 also provides data on activity levels over time for both still-married women and women who became widowed over a two-year interval. These data show unambiguously that widowed women were no different from still-married women in terms of overall activity level. These results correspond well to the results for morale. We found that morale dropped but not to a negative level that could be expected to result in depression, which in turn might have suppressed activity level. So the lack of decline in activity level among widows is indirect evidence of continued morale at a level that is at least adequate for normal functioning. In other words, even in the face of widowhood, women were able to adapt and continue their social functioning.

Although the number of just-widowed men was very small, 6 of the 12 (50%) reported a decline in activity level after widowhood, a much higher percentage than for just-widowed women (33.3%). This finding, coupled with the fact that just-widowed men showed a much higher proportion with sharp drops in morale compared with just-widowed women, suggests that men were much more likely to be affected negatively by widowhood compared with women.

Continuity theory would lead us to expect that widowed persons, being people with a long history of lifestyles built around being part of a married couple, would attempt to remarry. This is indeed the case for men. Of the 17 men who were widowed over the first five waves of the OLSAA, 12 eventually remarried. For women, however, the availability of potential marriage partners limits the opportunity for remarriage; of 46 women who became widowed over the first five waves, only 3 remarried.

However, the lack of marriage partners is not the only reason widowed persons may not seek remarriage. For a small minority, widowhood was a release from a no-longer desirable lifestyle, and the existence of a viable social role for widowed women (Lopata 1996) allows women who become widowed to embrace a lifestyle of living alone. In addition, widowhood for older women is akin to retirement in the sense that there is little cultural pressure to replace the former role. Retired people are not expected to seek another job, and older widows are not expected to find another spouse.

Our findings with regard to retirement and widowhood show that although retirement and widowhood are role changes that most definitely call for adaptation, most respondents were able to adapt to these changes and to maintain or improve their morale and activity level. But what about the beginnings of physical disability? Can older people adapt as easily to the onset of limitations in physical functioning?

Onset of Functional Limitations

The onset of limitations in physical functioning is a third type of change that is common to later adulthood and usually requires some degree of adaptation. In this section I first do a quantitative analysis of changes in functional capability comparable to the analyses I did earlier for retirement and widowhood. Then I move to a case history analysis to examine the forms of adaptation used by respondents who experienced a loss of functional capability.

Table 4.10 shows morale data over various waves of the OLSAA for respondents who retained high capability in physical functioning and those who experienced a drop from high physical functioning to being able to perform only three or fewer functions. As in the case of retirement and widowhood, the numbers of respondents who experienced declining functional capability were small in any single survey interval. But by combining data for two-year intervals, we were able to develop before-and-after data for 38 men and 29 women who experienced the onset of significant functional limitations during a two-year survey interval. Comparing their morale score patterns over time with morale score patterns for respondents who retained high functional capability over time, we see that there is no statistically significant difference between the two groups. Contrary to what we might expect, among men who experienced functional limitations, a *higher* percentage had increased morale (39.5%) compared with men who retained high functional capability (28% with increased morale), but the magnitude of this difference is well within the range of chance variation. On the other hand, women who experienced the onset of functional limitations were *less* likely to show an increase in morale (17.2%) compared with women still having high functioning (31.8%). However, because of the small number of women who experienced the onset of functional limitation, there is about a 10 percent probability that this difference is the result of chance.

Table 4.11 shows data for activity levels over time for the same two subgroups of respondents. There were no significant differences in patterns of

TABLE 4.10. Morale for those who retained physical function versus those who experienced onset of significant functional limitations over two-year intervals, by gender

	Morale					
	Increased		Unchanged		Decreased	
	N	%	N	%	N	%
High functioning T_1 and T_2						
Men ($N = 468$)	131	28.0	224	47.9	113	24.1
Women ($N = 402$)	128	31.8*	185	46.0	89	22.2
High functioning T_1 and three or more functional limitations T_2						
Men ($N = 38$)	15	39.5	16	42.1	7	18.4
Women ($N = 29$)	5	17.2*, **	16	55.2	8	27.6

* Gender differences significant at the .05 level (chi-square).
** Difference between high functioning and functional limitation groups significant for women at the .10 level (chi-square).

TABLE 4.11. Activity level for those who retained physical functioning versus those who experienced onset of significant functional limitations over two-year intervals, by gender

	Activity Level					
	Increased		Unchanged		Decreased	
	N	%	N	%	N	%
High functioning T_1 and T_2						
Men ($N = 477$)	69	14.5	277	58.1	131	27.5
Women ($N = 438$)	75	17.1	247	56.4	116	26.5
High functioning T_1 and three or more functional limitations T_2						
Men ($N = 37$)	5	13.5	25	67.6	7	18.6
Women ($N = 30$)	5	16.7	16	53.3	9	30.0

overall activity level between the still-high-functioning group and those who developed functional limitations. There were no significant gender differences either.

These data indicate that in the aggregate, people who experience the beginnings of physical disability are able to cope with these changes without significant negative effects on either morale or activity level. However, the aggregate data give us no way to explain how this adaptation occurs. To understand the dynamics of adaptation to the early onset of physical disability, I now turn to an analysis of the relationship between the onset of functional limitations and various components of the self.

Functional Limitation and the Self

In this section, I look at how functional disability[2] influences various components of the self: personal agency, emotional resilience, and personal goals. Because continuity theory is about long-term patterns of thought and behavior, the analyses presented here emphasize long time intervals, beginning with the relationships between antecedent and current social structural variables and perceived personal agency.

As shown in Table 4.12, respondents who scored high in personal agency were those who strongly agreed that they could do just about anything they put their mind to, could be called a go-getter, and if they wanted something they went out and got it. I use path analysis to look at age, gender, and education (as antecedent structural variables) and functional disability (as a

[2] Some restrict the term *disability* to mean the underlying physical cause of functional limitation, but here I use *disability* to refer to an inability to perform specific physical behavioral functions.

TABLE 4.12. Indicators of self-referent dimensions

Self-Referent Dimension	Specific Statements Used as Indicators
Personal agency	*Indicate how much you agree or disagree with each of the following statements as they apply to you now:* I can do just about anything I put my mind to. [agree] I am a go-getter. [agree] If I want something, I go out and get it. [agree]
Emotional resilience	*Next is a series of items about how life has been for you recently. Indicate how much you agree or disagree with each item:* Things keep getting worse as I get older. [disagree] Little things bother me more this year. [disagree] I sometimes think that life isn't worth living. [disagree] I am as happy now as when I was younger. [disagree] I have a lot to be sad about. [disagree] I am afraid of a lot of things. [disagree] I get mad more than I used to. [disagree] I take things hard. [disagree]
Personal goals	*Rate how important or unimportant each goal is in your life:* Being well-read and informed Having close ties with my family Being prominent in community affairs Having a substantial income Having a satisfying job Forming close, long-lasting friendships Being self-reliant Seeking new experiences and opportunities Having a comfortable place to live Being seen as a good person by others Being dependable and reliable Being a religious person

current, intervening social structural variable) as influences on perceptions of personal agency. I also include a baseline measure of personal agency.

Figure 4.1 shows the basic logic of the two-stage multiple regression analysis used to generate the path coefficients. In stage one, gender, age, and education were treated as exogenous social structural variables and used to predict functional disability (adjusted R^2 for this stage of the model was .316), with age, gender, and education all contributing to the prediction of 1991 functional disability.[3] This analysis provides an assessment of the indirect effects of social structural variables on personal agency through their effects on functional disability. In stage two, the direct effects of age, gender, and education on personal agency in 1991 were assessed. Baseline personal agency in 1981 was also included in the regression analysis. Functional dis-

---

[3] Data from 1991 were used to provide a larger number of respondents for the detailed analysis reported later in the chapter.

ability score in 1991 was taken as a concurrent social structural variable. Functional disability score was the number of everyday activities, such as working at a full-time job, walking a half-mile, doing heavy work around the house (such as shoveling snow or washing walls), walking up and down stairs, doing light housework, and getting out into the community, which the respondent reported being unable to do. The influence of antecedent social structural variables was evaluated in two ways: direct effects on 1991 personal agency scores and indirect effects through the impact of antecedent social structural characteristics on 1991 functional disability. The numbers by the lines in Figure 4.1 are the standardized regression coefficients for each link. For more straightforward presentation, statistically nonsignificant paths were omitted.

The results of this modest path analysis are interesting. First, continuity of personal agency is the most powerful factor operating in the model (beta = .492). Such stability of indicators over time is not unusual in gerontological research, which in itself could be taken as support for continuity theory. But note that the association of 1981 and 1991 personal agency scores is far from perfect. Continuity was the most powerful factor, but other factors operated as well. Second, neither age, nor education, nor gender had a direct effect on personal agency, either in 1981 or in 1991. This finding is certainly contrary to the conventional wisdom, which would lead us to expect lower personal

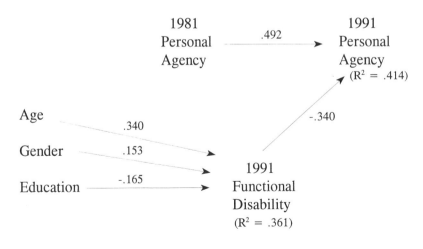

FIGURE 4.1. Path analysis of predictors of perceptions of personal agency.

agency scores from the older, the less-educated, and the female respondents. Third, age, education, and gender *all* had significant *indirect* effects on personal agency through their influence on functional disability. This finding supports the notion that antecedent social structural attributes have their impact indirectly, through their influence on the more immediate conditions confronting the aging self. Fourth, among social structural characteristics, functional disability was the only one that had a significant direct impact on personal agency (beta $= -.340$). This finding suggests that, compared with general social structural factors, socially conditioned physical constraints have a more powerful effect on perceived personal agency. I will return to this theme when I look in more detail at the effect of functional disability on various components of the self. The overall adjusted R^2 for the model predicting 1991 personal agency was .414, a respectable level of explanation from just two direct independent variables.

Theoretically, this analysis supports the idea that continuity in the personal agency component of the self is prevalent across a large variety of social structural subgroups within the aging population. But this correlation-based operational definition of continuity is unsatisfying because it does not get at the individual balance of continuity and change. To illustrate how this concern can be addressed, I next examine a small subsample in much greater detail.

Our second analysis looks separately at the effects of aging on the self compared with effects of functional disability on the self. Following continuity theory, the hypothesis is that people who age without disability show continuity in all three dimensions of the self, even though they might experience social structural changes such as retirement or widowhood. Following my argument on the potential negative effects of disability on the self, the hypothesis is that development of disability has greater potential negative effects on various dimensions of the self compared with aging (Atchley 1991). The rationale is that the development of disability alters the individual's social structural location in ways that introduce physical and lifestyle constraints on action, which in turn negatively influence people's perceptions of their personal agency, reduce their conceptions of themselves as emotionally resilient, and cause them to abandon some of their personal goals.

To assess the effects of both aging and disability adequately, it was desirable to be able to begin with a population that had no functional disabilities and then to compare continuity and discontinuity in self-conceptions over time for two groups: those who experienced aging as a gentle slope and those who developed several functional disabilities during the study. The disability group consisted of 29 respondents who reported no functional disabilities in

TABLE 4.13. Age and gender of disability and control group respondents in 1991

Age	Total	Female	Male
65–69	8	2	6
70–74	12	8	4
75–79	20	12	8
80–84	14	8	6
85–89	2	2	
90–94	2	2	
Total	58	34	24

1975 but who had developed three or more functional disabilities by 1991. Again, *functional disability* was defined as the inability to perform three or more of the following: work at a full-time job; heavy work around the house; ordinary work around the house; walk a half-mile; walk up and down stairs; and go out to a movie, to church, to a meeting, or to visit. A control group was constructed from among those who had no functional disabilities at any time during the study by matching respondents in the disability group with those in the control pool on age, gender, and education. This matching strategy was used because these social structural variables influenced personal agency indirectly in the earlier analysis. Controlling for them allows us to compare the disability and control groups without the muddying indirect effects of age, gender, and education. The final groups consisted of 29 respondents each — 17 women and 12 men in each group. Table 4.13 shows the age distribution of all respondents in both groups in 1991, by gender.

It is a difficult task to trace patterns of response on multiple indicators over five waves of data. The standard computer data analysis packages do not provide an option for displaying data this way, and there are no statistical procedures that allow what is in effect a multivariate time series analysis. Instead, worksheets were constructed which portrayed individual survey items or scale scores in each column, and the rows were the five survey waves. The investigator could then look down the columns and highlight the magnitude and direction of change that occurred over time for each item or scale score. Positive and negative changes were color coded separately. In addition to charting all of the self-referent items listed in Table 4.4, the worksheets included data over time on functional disabilities or lack of them, marital status, the interval in which retirement and or widowhood occurred (if applicable), level of participation over time in each of 16 types of activity, and overall activity level scores over time. Overall morale was not included because several of the morale scale items were used to measure the self-referent category of emotional resilience.

To aggregate data on personal agency, emotional resilience, and personal

TABLE 4.14. Decision criteria for classifying cases in terms of degree and direction of continuity and change, by self-referent dimension

Degree and Direction of Continuity and Change	Self-Referent Dimension		
	Personal Agency	Emotional Resilience	Personal Goals
Positive change	2+ increased	4+ increased	6+ increased
	1 or fewer consistent	4 or fewer consistent	6 or fewer consistent
Continuity with positive change	1/3 increased	2–3 increased	3–5 increased
	2/3 consistent	5–6 consistent	7–9 consistent
Continuity	3/3 consistent	7+ consistent	10+ consistent
Continuity with negative change	1/3 declined	2–3 declined	3–5 declined
	2/3 consistent	5–6 consistent	7–9 consistent
Negative change	2+ declined	4+ declined	6+ declined
	1 or fewer consistent	4 or fewer consistent	6 or fewer consistent

goals and to assess continuity and change within cases required the development of decision rules. For example, data on personal agency came from three indicators. If at least two of the three showed improvement over time and the other was consistent, then the case was classified as "positive change." If two of the three remained consistent over time and one improved, the case was classified as "continuity with positive change." If all indicators were consistent over time, the case was categorized as "continuity." If two indicators showed consistency over time and one showed negative change, then the case was classified as "continuity with negative change." If two or more indicators showed negative change over time and the other indicator showed continuity, then the case was classified as "negative change." Table 4.14 shows the decision rules used to classify cases into the three multiple-item self-referent categories by degree and direction of change or continuity.

To employ the scheme shown in Table 4.14 also required decision rules in terms of what was continuity. Obviously, continuity or consistency could be defined as having the same score over time, and many respondents showed this pattern on several items. However, the items all used a "strongly agree," "agree," "disagree," "strongly disagree" response format, so a more conceptual definition of what constituted continuity could be adopted easily. For example, suppose we look at the item "I can do just about anything I put my mind to" and a respondent scored "strongly agree," "agree," "strongly agree," "strongly agree," and "agree" over the five waves of the study. Is this change or continuity? There is fluctuation among the responses, but they remain in the "agree" category, so an argument can be made for consistency or continuity but not absolute stability. On the other hand, suppose another respondent to that same item checked "strongly agree," "agree," "strongly agree," "strongly agree," and *"disagree."* This latter respondent not only made a shift in magnitude of response from time 4 to time 5 but also switched from feeling able to "do just about anything I put my mind to" to not feeling that way. This is a clear-cut case of discontinuity. This approach was used to score the individual items in terms of continuity or change over time. When respondents switched from "agree" to "disagree" or vice versa from time to time over the study, they were classified as reporting change. Fluctuations *within* the "agree" or "disagree" category were classified as continuity. For the personal goals items, the major categories were "important" and "unimportant," with the strongest responses being labeled "very."

Table 4.15 shows the degree and direction of change and continuity for the three dimensions of the self, by disability status. Perhaps the most striking finding is that unadulterated continuity accounted for a majority of the cases for both the disability and control groups in five of the six analyses. Only personal agency for those who developed disability showed less than a majority (41%) in the continuity category. This is strong support for the assertion in continuity theory that people are predisposed to maintain consistent patterns of thinking about themselves as they adapt to aging. Note that these findings span multiple data points over a period of 16 years, and remember that disability and control group differences are not influenced by age, gender, or education because the groups were matched on these characteristics.

A second important finding is that the onset of disability influenced some self-referent dimensions but not others. Personal agency for those who developed disability is the only situation in which a substantial proportion (28%) experienced negative change. In addition, for emotional resilience, continuity with negative change is more prevalent in the disability group compared with the control group (38% compared with 21%). On the other hand, the self-values that comprise personal goals are completely dominated by unadulterated continuity for both disability and control groups.

We expected that the activity constraints of disability would reduce perceptions of personal agency. This expectation is partially borne out but only compared with the very low prevalence of negative change in the control group, which again supports the idea that aging in itself seldom has an effect on perceptions of personal agency. Only 28 percent of those who became disabled experienced negative change. A majority of those who developed disability showed either continuity or improvement in their sense of personal agency. The disability and control groups are not very different in terms of the proportions who experienced continuity with negative change in their perceptions of personal agency over time. This means, of course, that some

TABLE 4.15. Longitudinal continuity and change in dimensions of the self, by disability status

	Self-Referent Dimension											
	Personal Agency				Emotional Resilience				Personal Goals			
	No Disability		Developed Disability		No Disability		Developed Disability		No Disability		Developed Disability	
Degree and Direction of Continuity and Change	N	%	N	%	N	%	N	%	N	%	N	%
Positive change	1	3	1	3	1	3	1	3			3	10
Continuity with positive change	4	14	2	7	2	7	15	52	28	97	24	83
Continuity	15	52	12	41	20	66	11	38	1	3	2	7
Continuity with negative change	7	24	6	21	6	21	2	7				
Negative change	2	7	8	28*	1	3						
Total	29	100	29	100	29	100	29	100	29	100	29	100

[a] Group difference significant at the .05 level, using chi-square.

negative change occurred even among those who experience physical aging as a gentle slope. Positive change in personal agency is rare for either group.

We expected that the frustrations of disability would result in decreased emotional resilience, but a very large majority of both groups experienced continuity or positive change in perceived emotional resilience.

We expected that the realities of functional disability would cause the individuals in the disability group to downgrade the importance of some personal goals, but personal goals showed a very high prevalence of continuity. Regardless of disability status, people tended to maintain their personal goals over time. The individuals in this study had very different priorities in terms of ratings of their personal goals. For example, 37 respondents thought that "being a religious person" was important; 21 thought this goal was unimportant. There was considerable variety among individuals in value profiles, but there was very little intraindividual change in values over time.

To get a sense of the dynamics of negative change in self-perceptions, we looked closely at the cases in which such changes occurred. In the cases that involved disability, the dynamics of declining perceptions of personal agency were straightforward. In nearly all of the eight cases of negative change in personal agency after disability, the respondents had experienced profound lifestyle changes. For example, these respondents reported the onset of serious and highly constraining underlying conditions such as emphysema, severe asthma, chronic bronchitis, acute leukemia, Parkinson disease, and paralysis. Their negative views of their personal agency were highly realistic in view of the activity restrictions imposed on them by their chronic conditions.

The two control group respondents who showed negative change in their perceptions of personal agency were men in their early 80s who experienced dramatic activity losses in key activities. Specifically, having given up long-time participation in sports characterized both of the respondents in the control group who had a negative change in their perceptions of personal agency. One also reported a substantial reduction in his frequency of church attendance. Thus, significant reductions in specific role-related activity, not generalized changes such as retirement, were associated with negative changes in personal agency for these two control group men who reported negative change in the absence of functional disability.

These findings have several implications for the study of the aging self. Although the small size of the samples poses a serious limit on the generalizability of the findings, the results do suggest several theoretical and methodological points that might be worth taking into account in future research.

First, personal agency, emotional resilience, and personal goals appear to be separate dimensions of the self, and these separate dimensions showed different patterns of continuity and change over time. Personal goals fluctuated very little over time and, contrary to expectations, did not shift to accommodate disability or decline in the frequency of specific day-to-day activities. Another way of saying this is that although middle-aged and older individuals vary considerably in terms of what they think is important, once they develop a personal value system, they tend to retain that value system even in the face of substantial external change.

Emotional resilience also showed a high degree of continuity over time, but disability introduced negative elements into that continuity much more frequently than mere aging did. Finally, among elders who developed disability a substantial minority experienced negative change in their perceptions of their personal agency. Disabled elders who showed a declining sense of agency were quite likely to be dealing with very limiting underlying conditions such as breathing disorders, paralysis, leukemia, or Parkinson disease. Elders whose disabilities consisted of less profoundly disabling conditions such as arthritis, musculoskeletal problems, or even low vision were more likely to report continuity in their sense of personal agency.

At least for the dimensions of the self reported here, there was much more continuity than change in self-referent conceptions over a considerable length of time. These findings suggest that the internal desire for continuity overrides external, situational pressures to change, at least for these three elements of the self. Thus, the propensity toward continuity might be seen as establishing a threshold that could be used to identify when the dynamic model of the self of Markus and Herzog (1991) might be mobilized into action. In other words, continuity could be expected to be the general rule, but when change exceeds a subjectively defined threshold, then changes in the self might be expected.

In the absence of seriously limiting disability, aging people achieve continuity across various dimensions of the self, which supports continuity theory. Seriously limiting disability tended to supersede the continuity principle for a small minority of respondents, but only for personal agency. Less serious disability and reductions in longstanding activities can bring a negative tone to continuity without neutralizing its value as a concept that describes the patterns of self-perception over time.

In later life, functional limitations often occur gradually. Although some conditions such a stroke or injury can produce profound and sudden disability, more often chronic conditions, functional limitations, and disabilities develop over a considerable length of time. Studies of disability in the aging population have tended to focus on the *outcomes* of the disablement process, particularly disability in Activities of Daily Living (ADLs), rather than on the evolution of disability over time (Verbrugge and Jette 1994). But understanding the antecedents, progression, and consequences of disability requires a longer view. Chronic conditions have social antecedents such as lifestyle risk factors, and individuals do not simply sit idly by and observe the erosion of their capacity for independent living. They often actively adapt and compensate to minimize the effects of chronic conditions and functional limitations. Very little research in gerontology has looked at the active adaptive response of elders to either sudden or gradual onset of chronic illness and functional limitation (Becker 1993). Next I consider how people adapt their activities in response to the onset of functional limitations.

Several conceptual perspectives can be used to look at the relationships among functional limitations, disability in activities, and subjective well-being in aging people. Activity substitution (Havighurst 1963; Rosow 1967; Mannell 1993), consolidation (Atchley 1985), continuity (Atchley 1989, 1995), and disengagement (Cumming and Henry 1961; Johnson and Barer 1992) are all conceptualizations that can be used to look at adaptation to changes that threaten to create or actually cause role or activity losses.

Activity theory is a homeostatic equilibrium theory. It presumes that individuals are motivated to cope with losses by restoring the previous equilibrium (Rosow 1967). The initial equilibrium in activities could be at any overall level of activity ranging from high to low. The early statements of activity theory presumed that *substitution* of new activities for lost activities was the primary means of adapting to role loss. This mechanistic conception is tied to a highly positional or structural view of roles. A second type of equilibrium theory presumed *consolidation* (Atchley 1985), that people cope with role losses by consolidating their activity patterns and redistributing their energies to the remaining roles. In this style of coping with role loss, equilibrium is restored by increasing the level of participation for those activities that remain in order to maintain an initial overall activity level. Thus, the pattern of activities is altered, but the overall activity level is maintained. This conception presumes individual agency and internal motivation. *Continuity theory* (Atchley 1989) assumes that individuals avoid or minimize the effects of role loss by maintaining their longstanding structures of activity. Continuity theory assumes that people who cannot avoid role loss or constraints on customary role behavior try to preserve the *pattern* of activity but cope with functional limitations by reducing the overall *level* of participation. This approach could accommodate a decline in overall activity level but would

TABLE 4.16. Theories of coping with activity loss and effects on subjective well-being

	Maintain Activity Equilibrium			Moderate Activity Decline	Profound Activity Decline
	Continuity	Substitution	Consolidation	Continuity	Disengagement
Activity implications	Both pattern and level maintained	Losses offset by new activities, level maintained	Level maintained but fewer activities	Maintain pattern but level declines	Number of activities reduced sharply and overall activity level declines sharply
Negative effect on subjective well-being	None	None	Moderate	Moderate	Severe

retain the general pattern. *Disengagement theory* (Johnson and Barer 1992) involves a fundamental change in both pattern and level of activity. Individuals who disengage drop a large number of their previously customary activities entirely, and their overall activity level also drops dramatically. Lost activities are not replaced, and activities are rarely increased to offset losses. For the disengaged person very little of their predisengagement lifestyle remains.

These conceptions all rely on assumptions about the underlying motivation of individuals who are coping with change. All but disengagement theory assume that people want to maintain their level or pattern of activity or both. The reasoning here is that people want to preserve linkages with their past patterns, which are presumed to have been comfortable ones. The underlying internal motivations linked to disengagement have included increasing preference for introspection (Cumming and Henry 1961), a desire to conserve energy (Johnson and Barer 1992), and a recognition that options for replacing lost activities or restoring previous activity levels are limited (Atchley 1985). The literature on disengagement theory also indicates that people can be forced into disengagement by the lack of opportunity that results from age discrimination or from the social structure of access to opportunities (Roman and Taietz 1967; Carp 1968). It could also be broadened to include constraints stemming from discrimination against those with disabilities (Luborsky 1994).

Ideas concerning the impact of activity loss on subjective well-being again focus on equilibrium, continuity, and disengagement. The theories listed above suggest that both pattern and level of participation are important. Table 4.16 summarizes the conceptual links among changes in activity patterns and levels, various conceptions of adaptation, and expected outcomes in terms of subjective well-being. We would expect that maintaining an equilibrium that preserved both the number of activities and activity level (continuity or substitution) would have little negative effect on subjective well-being. A middle position that preserved the customary activity pattern but with a lower level of activity (decline with continuity) or preserved activity level but with fewer activities (consolidation) might be expected to cause a mild sense of loss and therefore have a moderate negative effect on subjective well-being. Continuity theory would lead us to predict that disengagement would *not* occur in the absence of profound constraints, and we would expect disengagement to have a strong negative effect on subjective well-being. If, on the other hand, there is intrinsic motivation for disengagement, then disengagement might be expected to have less profound effects on subjective well-being.

The present analysis uses the disability and control groups described above to study the relationship between the development of functional limitations and the adaptation of activities over a period of 16 years. It also examines the consequences for subjective well-being of adopting various activity patterns in response to functional limitations.

Functional limitation was measured by the six-item scale described previously. These items formed a near-perfect Guttman Scale pattern (coefficient of reproducibility = .97). Those individuals who could *not* perform three of the listed activities were highly likely *not* to be able to work full-time, do heavy work around the house, and walk a half-mile. Those with four functional limitations generally lost the ability to walk up and down stairs, those with five lost the ability to do ordinary work around the house, and getting out into the community was usually the last function lost. By 1991, 10 of the functional limitation group had lost three functions, 13 had lost four functions, 5 had lost five functions, and only 1 had lost all six functions.

In addition, open-ended questions provided information about specific favorite activities that were constrained by functional limitation as well as the underlying causes of those limitations, usually chronic conditions or permanent injuries. Respondents also occasionally wrote amplifying comments on the questionnaires that could be used to interpret their situations further.

This analysis can best be described as a qualitative analysis of mostly quantitative data. The same longitudinal worksheets used in the previous analysis were used here, but the data were analyzed in the form of individual longitudinal case histories. Although each of the activity patterns is unique, the respondents could be classified into one of six categories based on the relative stability of activity level and pattern over the duration of the study. Respondents with overall equilibrium in activity level were in the *continuity* category, which showed little change in either level or pattern of activity; or in the *consolidation* category, which showed equilibrium in overall activity level (high, moderate, or low) but change in the pattern of activity as a result of increasing some activities to offset declines in others. Those in the *decline with continuity* category showed a decline in overall activity level but consistency over time in their pattern of activity. Respondents in the *disengagement* category showed a sharp reduction in the number of activities, very little or no increase to offset activity losses, and a large decline in overall activity level. With the exception of *substitution*, which was not observed in any of the cases, these categories match the types based on the theoretical literature summarized in Table 4.16. In addition, there was an additional category: respondents who showed a decline in overall activity level but with some offsetting increases in a few activities (labeled *decline with some offsets*).

Results are presented in two parts: (1) case histories showing the dynamics of the relationship between the development of functional limitation and activity adaptation patterns, and (2) a comparison of patterns of activity adaptation in the group who developed disabilities with patterns of activity adaptation in the control group.

Patterns of Coping with Functional Limitations

Selected case records provide a sense of the dynamics associated with various outcomes. Details of the case histories have been altered slightly in some cases to preserve anonymity of the respondents. Here I focus on cases that illustrate how the development of functional limitations relates to activity adaptation and subjective well-being. First I look at cases that illustrate the *consolidation* category.

Ned was 81 at the time of the 1991 survey. A well-educated schoolteacher who retired in 1980, he and his wife had lived in the community for more than 40 years by 1991. Their income put them solidly in the middle class among retirees. Ned had already experienced two functional limitations by the time he retired, and by 1991 he only retained the capacity to get out into the community. He was partially paralyzed, used a walker, and gave up driving after 1981. Ned had never engaged in a large number of activities. In 1975, he participated in only 8 of the 18 activity types listed in the OLSAA questionnaire; however, he maintained his participation in nearly all of his customary activities, particularly going to plays and concerts, traveling, reading, being with his many friends, and spending time with his family. His paralysis caused him to give up gardening, which he had done occasionally; he no longer went to ballgames, and he was no longer involved in the local teachers association, but he offset these losses by increasing his involvement in community organizations considerably and spending more time watching television. Ned was a contented man in 1991. He saw himself realistically as less mobile than he was when he could walk unassisted and drive, but his morale was above the average for the entire panel.

June is on the opposite end of the continuum from Ned. She experienced less severe loss of function and was able to maintain a very high level of activity by increasing some activities to offset losses of others. June retired from her clerical job at the age of 67, and she and her husband enjoyed a modest income. In 1975, June participated to at least some extent in every activity listed in the questionnaire, and she maintained that distinction through 1991, despite having three functional limitations. Her cutbacks in gardening, political activity, and attending church functions were offset by increases in walking, attending concerts and going to movies, and involvement in community organizations. Although she was able to maintain a very high level of activity into her middle 70s and her morale remained stable, June felt sad that her life was not as full as she would like it to be, which was a new attitude associated with her experience of functional limitations. This suggests that for June, maintaining the quantity of activity is not the same as maintaining the quality of activity.

Walter was 79 in 1991, and he had retired from his job as a janitor at the age of 64. He and his wife had a very modest income. Walter experienced a substantial decrease in functional abilities, but he could maintain his activities at a relatively stable level. Between 1979 and 1981, he went from being able to perform all six functions to only being able to get out into the community. He received personal assistance from both his wife and a paid helper. Despite his arthritis, Walter was able to continue his frequent participation in gardening, woodworking, reading, church activities, playing cards, and spending time with friends. His only activity losses were in his labor union involvement and being with his family, both of which he continued to do less frequently. He offset these losses by increasing his interest and participation in a variety of spectator sports, especially local baseball and softball, and in community organizations. Despite his many functional difficulties, Walter maintained a stable and positive attitude toward his life.

Doris experienced hip problems that caused her to abandon many of her customary activities, but she maintained her level of activity by increasing her participation in already familiar ones. Doris worked as a physical education teacher until her retirement at age 63. At the time of the 1991 survey, she was 79. In 1975 the only activity she did not participate in was being with children because she had never married and was childless. But by 1977, joint problems had caused her to experience two functional limitations, and by 1979 she had experienced three. Surgery brought her back to all functions but full-time employment by 1981, but by 1991 she had returned to having three functional limitations. Doris went from often participating in sports to not participating at all. She also stopped participating in a bridge group, in the teachers association, and in politics. She increased her frequency of going to plays and concerts, participation in community organizations, attending sporting events, and attending church. In 1991, Doris had a very positive attitude about her retirement and above-average morale.

Betty was a widow throughout the study. By 1991 she was 86 and had lived in the community all of her life. She had never been employed, and her only income was a modest Social Security survivor benefit, which put her in a low-income category. She did not report significant functional limitations until the 1991 survey, when she showed four of them, which she attributed to a heart condition. She received personal assistance from her children. She was not particularly active even when she had full functional capability, and in 1975 there were only four activities that she did often: gardening, spending time with children and grandchildren, reading, and watching television. She still did those things in 1991, although at a slightly lower frequency for gardening and being with family and a slightly higher frequency for reading. The activities she dropped—attending social events, attending church, and participating in community organizations and political activities — were things she did only occasionally in 1975. Betty had a positive attitude toward herself and her life, but from 1981 to 1991 her morale dropped from average to below average for the panel.

These cases illustrate that whether functional limitations are severe or moderate and whether initial activity level is high, moderate, or low, respondents were able to maintain their activity levels by substituting increased participation in familiar activities for losses in activities resulting from functional limitations. The overwhelming majority of these respondents had morale that was average or higher and a positive attitude toward retirement. These data support the idea that consolidation is usually a satisfying pattern for those who are able to achieve it.

| | | | | |

The *decline with continuity* category is made up of respondents who experienced sharp increases in functional limitations and sharp reductions in activity levels but who were also able to maintain their participation in a wide variety of customary activities.

Thelma was 77 in 1991. She lived with her husband and reported a very modest income. She had a heart condition that caused her mild functional limitations through 1981, but by 1991 she reported four functional limitations. Thelma was very active in 1975 and participated often or very often in 10 of the 18 activity areas. Her favorites were gardening, writing, handiwork, and being with friends and family. By 1991, she had managed to maintain participation in all 10 of her primary activities but at a much reduced level. She did not offset these losses by increasing her involvement in other activities. Thelma enjoyed above-average morale for the first four waves of the study, but by 1991 it had dropped to below average. However, from 1981 to 1991, her concept of herself remained stable and very positive. She still saw herself as active, involved, and very busy, even though her objective activity level score had dropped from 87 to 65. Although she experienced a substantial reduction in activity, she was still a relatively active person in 1991, with an activity score still above the overall panel mean.

In 1991, Ruth was 74, had been widowed for 12 years, and was a retired public school teacher with relatively high retirement income. She experienced a drop from an average activity level in 1975 to a low activity level in 1991. Her functional limitations were the result of a hip condition that began to pose problems as early as 1977. She received personal assistance from a home care worker. By 1991, she was still able to attend church or social functions, but she could not perform any of the other five functions. In 1975, she often engaged in 10 of the 18 activity categories, her favorite activity being gardening. By 1991, she had given up participating in games and in the teachers association. She had reduced her level of participation in spectator art, handiwork, and travel. She partially offset these declines by attending church functions much more frequently, and she maintained a high level of participation in gardening, being with family and friends, reading, and watching television. Thus, although Ruth's activity level dropped substantially from 1975 to 1991, she managed to maintain participation in all but two of the activities that she did often. As a result of her substantial drop in activity, she saw herself as quite uninvolved and idle in 1991 compared with her self-concept as quite involved and busy in in 1975. However, she remained satisfied with her life, and her morale was about average for the overall panel.

These cases indicate that respondents who encounter substantial loss of functions and corresponding reductions in activity are able to maintain a positive mental outlook if they can remain at least partially involved in their customary activities.

| | | | | |

The *decline with some offsetting increases* category was made up of respondents who reported an overall decline in activity level and a loss of customary activity categories but also increases in a few activities to partially offset the declines in others.

Vera never married and was 79 in 1991. She had been retired throughout the study. She developed mobility problems in 1979 because of a hip condition, and she continued to have three functional limitations in 1991. As a result of them, she gave up gardening and playing golf completely, which reduced her overall activity level a modest amount. She partially offset these changes by slightly increasing her participation in community service organizations, church, and spectator sports. She continued to see herself as an active and capable person, and her morale remained high and stable over the duration of the study.

Martha was 58 and married at the beginning of the study. Her activity level was moderate, and she engaged in most of the activity types. She developed a hip condition that caused three functional limitations in 1977. In 1979 her husband died. By 1991, she could still get out into the community but was unable to do any of the other functional tasks. Her overall activity level dropped from a moderate level in 1975 to a low level in 1991. She reduced her participation in knitting, playing cards, and in community service organizations substantially. She partially offset these declines by increasing her involvement in church and political activities. Although three of her close friends died between 1979 and 1991, she maintained frequent contact with those who remained. Her morale was average at the beginning of the study, dropped when her husband died in 1979, but came back up to average again in 1981. As late as 1979, she saw herself as active, involved, able, and satisfied. But by 1991, she saw herself as unhealthy, uninvolved, and idle. However, she remained satisfied with her life overall.

Even for those who were not able to offset declines in activity or maintain their basic pattern of activities, declines in activity did not tend to produce a drop in morale if the respondent was able to offset activity declines with increases at least partially. The key factor here seems to be that being able to adapt by taking action at least to some extent preserved the respondent's perception of personal agency. For example, both of the respondents described above continued to believe that they had the capacity to accomplish what they set out to do and to meet their own needs when they arose.

| | | | | |

The *disengagement* category consists of respondents who stopped participating in a large number of their customary activities. This category is based on the idea that functional limitation can cause people to abandon their usual activities and not replace them, which in turn can lead to sharply lower activity levels and in turn to lower morale. Disengagement is assumed to be the result of functional limitation rather than individual choice.

A never-employed housewife, Frances had asthma that began to limit her activities between 1975 and 1977. By 1991 Frances was 78 and had four functional limitations. She received help from an adult child, and she provided help to her husband. In 1975 her activity level was high, but her progressively disabling illness gradually caused her to abandon her participation in handicrafts, antique collecting, spectator sports, political activities, and community service organizations, social events, and church functions. She was only able to offset these substantial losses with modest increases in being with friends and reading. She went from having 3 activity areas in which she never participated in 1975 to 13 in 1991, a net loss of 10. Her general attitude about the quality of her life went from very positive to just barely positive. The onset of her asthma shifted her self-image from a concept of herself as someone who was healthy, involved, happy, hopeful, and busy to a someone who was sick, inactive, uninvolved, hopeless, sad, dissatisfied, and idle.

Charles spent more than 50 years as a sheet metal worker until he retired at age 71. He was 80 in 1991. Between 1981 and 1991, he went from having no functional limitations to having five. Never a very active man, Charles went from participating in just 10 of the 18 activity areas in 1975 to only 3 in 1991. He still sometimes spent time with his family, watched television often, and sometimes engaged in sporting activities. He stopped gardening, metal working, playing cards, attending sporting events, traveling, spending time with friends, reading, and going to church. Yet Charles's morale score in 1991 was only slightly below average for the entire panel. He seems to have accepted his disengagement with reasonable equanimity, which may explain why he disengaged — it was okay with him. But he did not disengage simply as a function of growing older, he did so in tandem with the development of severe functional limitations.

Lyle was 71 in 1991. He had been a lawyer until his retirement in 1985, and his income was among the highest in the study. He had emphysema, which severely restricted his activities in 1991. He received personal assistance from his wife. He went from having one of the highest activity levels in the study in 1975 to having a low activity level in 1991. The number of activity areas he never participated in went from one to ten. The only activities he did often in 1991 were reading, being with friends and family, and watching television. He sometimes played cards, and he attended occasional social functions. The effect of his illness and the resulting functional limitations and activity disabilities on his attitudes was startling. As late as 1981, he was very positive about himself and his life. But by 1991, his morale was among the lowest in the study, and he saw himself as sick, inactive, immobile, unable, dependent, and idle and his life as empty. Obviously, Lyle was not happy with disengagement and did not go into it voluntarily.

In the control group we do not see evidence of disengagement from activities that compares even remotely with the substantial number of activity losses experienced by the disengagement category within the functional limitation group. For all of these respondents, disengagement followed or paralleled the development of substantial functional limitations. The outcome of disengagement in activities varied. Some respondents were able to maintain positive attitudes toward themselves and their lives, but most were not. These data show that being forced to disengage by functional limitations can produce very negative effects on subjective well-being. The aspect of subjective well-being that declines most frequently in response to increased functional limitation and activity disengagement is the sense of personal agency. Those who are forced to disengage by functional limitations feel that they are severely constrained in being able to make things happen. This pattern of change in personal agency did not occur in the other categories of response to functional limitation, nor did it occur in the control group.

Comparisons with Activity Adaptations in the Control Group

Now I compare activity adaptations between the group that developed functional limitations and the control group. Table 4.17 shows the distribution of cases by type of adaptation pattern for the functional limitation and

TABLE 4.17. Activity patterns for functional limitation and control groups

Activity Pattern	Functional Limitation Group		Control Group	
	N	%[a]	N	%[a]
Equilibrium				
Continuity			5	17.2
Substitution				
Consolidation	12	41.4	13	44.8
High	3		2	
Medium	6		9	
Low	3		2	
Decline with continuity	6	20.7	6	20.7
Disengagement	6	20.7*	1	3.4
Decline with some offsets	5	17.2	4	13.8
Total	29	100.0	29	99.9

[a] Rows do not add to 100 percent because of rounding.
* Chi-square difference significant at the .05 level.

control groups. *Continuity* in both pattern and level of activities was observed in only five cases, all of them in the control group. Two of these respondents maintained their pattern of activity and *increased* their overall activity level over the time of the study. *Consolidation* was the most common pattern in both groups, and there was no significant intergroup difference in the proportion showing this pattern. Likewise, about one fifth of each group fell into the *decline with continuity* pattern, and about one sixth of each group fell into the *decline with some offsets* category. However, the proportion showing *disengagement* was significantly greater in the functional limitation group (20.7%) compared with the control group (3.4%).

Not experiencing functional limitations allowed some members of the control group to keep their activity lifestyles intact. No one in the functional limitation group could do so, but many of them were able to use consolidation to maintain their overall activity level effectively. Disengagement occurred almost exclusively among the functional limitation group. The single case of disengagement in the control group was a 76-year-old woman whose husband was disabled and being cared for by her. Thus, caregiving responsibilities can cause activity disengagement. These findings strongly suggest that disengagement is not voluntary but results from the constraints imposed by one's own disability or by caregiving responsibilities.

Nevertheless, nearly two thirds of both groups showed activity patterns that preserved either the level or pattern of activity. In other words, most respondents who developed functional limitations were able to adapt their activities to achieve results similar to those for the control group, as continuity theory would lead us to expect.

Table 4.18 cross-classifies trends in activities by trends in morale for the

TABLE 4.18. Trend in morale by trend in activity for functional limitation and control groups

Trend in Activity	Trend in Morale			
	Increase	Stable	Small Decline	Large Decline
Functional limitation group				
Consolidation	2	5	2	3
Decline with continuity		4	2	
Decline with offsets		3	1	1
Disengagement		2		4
Total N	2	14	5	8
Total %	6.9	48.3	17.2	27.6
Control group				
Continuity	3	2		
Consolidation	2	11		
Decline with continuity		6		
Decline with offsets		4		
Disengagement				1
Total N	5	23		1
Total %[a]	17.2	79.3		3.4

[a] Row does not add to 100 percent because of rounding.

functional limitation group and the control group. Although a small majority of those who experienced three or more functional limitations reported stable or increased morale over time, a large minority (44.6%) experienced declining morale. This is in marked contrast with the control group, where all but one respondent reported stable or increased morale. (The older woman who experienced disengagement associated with caregiving responsibilities was the only control group respondent reporting declining morale.) These data indicate that although various adaptive patterns such as consolidation, declines with continuity, and declines with some offsets result in stable or increased morale for a majority of those who use these strategies, declines in morale were reported by a small number of functional limitation group respondents in each of these adaptive categories. And in the disengagement category, large declines in morale outnumbered stability by more than two to one. Thus, adaptive strategies that involve reorganizing activities in response to functional limitation are more effective at preserving activity pattern or level than in preventing declines in morale.

Understanding Activity Adaptations to the Onset of Functional Limitations

In terms of the expectations presented in Table 4.16, the substitution strategy did not occur in either group. Continuity of both activity pattern and activity level occurred only in the control group, as might be expected, and continuity was associated with stable or increased morale.

We expected that a reduction in either the number of activities (consolidation) or overall activity level (continuity with decline) might produce a sense of loss and therefore have a modest negative effect on morale. However, in the control group, neither of these patterns was associated with declines in morale. In the functional limitation group, on the other hand, there were cases of declining morale associated with consolidation or decline with continuity, but declining morale occurred in only a minority of cases even in the functional limitation group. Thus, being able to adapt, even if imperfectly, was associated with a greater likelihood of preserving morale rather than with experiencing a decline in morale even for those with functional limitations. But, as expected, disengagement was associated with a sharp decline in subjective well-being for five of the seven respondents who experienced disengagement.

This exploratory, qualitative analysis of longitudinal panel respondents looked at patterns of activity adaptation in response to the development of functional limitations. Because it dealt with activity changes primarily in community and leisure roles rather than in more basic activities required for adult independence, this study focused more on the beginnings of adaptation to disability rather than on coping with more basic changes. Indeed, none of the functional limitation group had any ADL disabilities, and only one had IADL (Instrumental Activities of Daily Living) disability, she needed help with meal preparation and managing money.

Several conceptions of adaptation to role loss were used to develop categories of adaptation to functional limitation. Each category represented a pathway of adaptation, and the study focused on what circumstances seemed to lead people to these various pathways with what consequences for subjective well-being.

Early versions of activity theory predicted that adaptation to role loss takes the form of maintaining equilibrium by substituting new activities for lost ones. Substitution was not found among those who developed functional limitations over the course of the study, nor was it observed in the control group. Respondents in this study rarely took up new activities in later life. (There was only one instance of a respondent taking up an entirely new type of activity; he was a functional limitation group respondent who began participating in a community service organization for the first time after his retirement.) Instead, equilibrium was maintained by continuing already existing activities, but this type of continuity occurred only in the control group. It was primarily a pattern of continuity rather than adapting to role loss.

When people reduced activities or dropped them, they usually adapted by increasing their involvement in those activities that remained. This consolidation approach was the most common pattern in terms of trends in activities. More than 40 percent of both the functional limitation group and the control group maintained relatively stable overall activity levels by increasing already existing activities to offset declines in other activities. Because this pattern is as common in the control group as in the functional limitation group, it appears to be a general pattern of adaptation to aging rather than a pattern specific to disability. Consolidation was associated with stable or increased subjective well-being in the control group, but in the functional limitation group consolidation did not provide protection from declining morale. Slightly more than 40 percent of the functional limitation group that was able to achieve consolidation still reported declines in morale, some of them substantial.

When we looked at how the development of functional limitations influenced various components of self-perception — personal agency, emotional resilience, and personal goals — the major impact of disability on the self was through its effect on one's conception of personal agency, with 28 percent of the disability group experiencing a negative change in their perception of personal agency, which was directly correlated with a decline in morale. Only 7 percent of the control group experienced a negative change in their perceived personal agency. The association between perceived personal agency and overall subjective well-being needs to be explored further.

Continuity theory predicts that in adapting to change, people attempt to preserve links to their past patterns of activity even if they cannot maintain equilibrium. About one fifth of both functional limitation and control groups fit this pattern. They experienced an overall decline in activity level but preserved the longstanding basic pattern of activities they reported throughout the study. Again, this would appear to be a path of adaptation to aging in general rather than an adaptation specific to functional limitation. This pattern is associated with continuity of morale in the control group and continuity or small declines in morale in the functional limitation group.

Empirically we observed a category that was not predicted by the various existing conceptions of adaptation to role loss. Decline in both number of activities and overall activity level with some offsetting activity increases was observed in about one sixth of both functional limitation and control group respondents. The best interpretation of this pathway seems to be that it is a response to aging, not just functional limitation, and it is an attempt to adapt to the greatest extent possible within the field created by the initial pattern of activities. This category was similar to the decline with continuity category in terms of effects on subjective well-being: stable for the control group and stability or small declines for all but one in the functional limitation group.

Disengagement theory predicts that some elders give up their activities voluntarily in order to conserve energy (Johnson and Barer 1992), and others are forced to disengage by physical or social constraints (Sill 1980; Roman and Taietz 1967). All of the cases of profound decline in both number and level of activities were either directly or indirectly related to functional limitation. The one control group respondent who disengaged did so in conjunction with caregiving responsibilities for her ADL-disabled husband. Of the seven respondents who showed activity disengagement, five showed a large decline in reported subjective well-being, and two showed stable subjective well-being. These data suggest that functional limitations and activity disengagement tend to have a negative effect on subjective well-being, which supports the predictions of those who theorized about the effects of involuntary disengagement. No cases of voluntary disengagement were observed in this study, but only 6 of our 58 respondents were age 85 or over, the category in which Johnson and Barer (1992) predicted voluntary disengagement.

These findings show the value of looking at detailed case data accumulated over time. This approach to data organization allows the investigator to see patterns and relationships within case records that can be used to classify respondents into categories of consistency or change over time. It also allows the investigator to take into account the order in which changes occur across dimensions. Its major limitation is that it requires detailed decision rules for issues such as stability and change. But because the data are mostly quantitative, once decision rules are agreed upon, the reliability of the classifications that result is quite high. However, an added disadvantage of this method is that it is very labor intensive and therefore practical mainly for studies with modest numbers of respondents.

The results show clearly the value of using competing conceptualizations within the same analysis. For example, had we only used the substitution hypothesis, we would have gotten disappointing results. But by including several other possibilities, we came away with a preliminary understanding of the limited conditions under which equilibrium models apply. We also could see that in reality the equilibria observed in level and pattern more nearly fit continuity and consolidation concepts than they did the early substitution concepts of activity theory because the activity substitution predicted by activity theory did not occur as a pattern. Likewise, we found that activity disengagement occurred primarily in response to functional limitations and usually had negative effects on subjective well-being. However, the most prevalent patterns typify adaptation to aging in general: consolidation, decline with continuity, and decline with some offsets. A next important step is to try out these ideas on other longitudinal data sets.

General Patterns of Adaptation

The previous analyses dissected adaptation in various ways to improve our understanding of specific ways in which people adapt. Next, I turn to a more holistic perspective that considers case examples of three major types of overall adaptation observed in the OLSAA: aging as a gentle slope, substantial change with positive outcome, and discontinuity with negative outcome.

Aging as a Gentle Slope

As we have seen over and over in this chapter, for most respondents in the OLSAA aging has been a gentle slope punctuated by changes that can be assimilated within a continuity framework relatively easily. Even the onset of functional limitation, because it does not usually require the substantial lifestyle changes that often accompany severe ADL dependence, is managed effectively using continuity of self and the customary pattern of lifestyle activities. As a gentle slope, aging does not result in lessened life satisfaction or an unwanted reduction in lifestyle activities.

> Gordon in many ways fit the stereotype of the "successful" retiree. He made the transition from middle age to later maturity with very little change and thus had no need for major life adjustments. Physically, mentally, and socially, aging had not imposed any limitation on his customary lifestyle. He remained in very good health, had very high morale and self-confidence, continued his customary patterns of activity, was happily married, continued to live in the same house, and enjoyed a very comfortable level of income throughout the study.
>
> Gordon was in his early 50s in 1975 and his early 70s in 1995. He and his wife launched the last of their four children into adulthood when he was in his early 60s. At age 65 he retired from his position as a middle-level executive for a large company. Although he liked his work very much and felt a great deal of accomplishment from it, he did not miss it. He felt that he had achieved his occupational goals and was ready to move on.
>
> In Gordon's eyes, child launching and retirement improved the quality of his already strong marriage by giving the couple more time alone to enjoy one another and to travel. In addition, he continued to visit with his children very often, as they lived in nearby cities. Thus, he was able to pass through these transitions with

either no change or an improvement in the relationships that formed an important part of his lifestyle.

After retirement, Gordon occupied himself by working around the house and engaging in a variety of physical activities, particularly golf in the summer and racquetball and swimming in the winter. He reported no difficulty whatever in "keeping myself productively busy." However, he did cut back substantially in his involvement in professional organizations after he retired.

Gordon's smooth transition into later life did not occur by accident. His good health was in part related to the fact that he intentionally led a health-promoting lifestyle; he scored well above average on our preventive health practices scale. In addition, he had a strong sense of life direction centered on keeping himself active and healthy and paying attention to his family and their needs. He also scored high in gerotranscendence—he felt that his inner life had become more important, he felt less fear of death, and he felt a greater connection to the universe.

Sally also experienced aging as a gentle slope, but in her case the transition was from later maturity to old age. Sally was already retired and in her very late 60s when our study began, and she was in her very late 80s in 1995. Throughout our study she scored very high in morale, rating of life in retirement, and self-confidence. Her overall activity level was high in 1975 and remained at that level in 1995. Her health remained very good throughout, and she reported no activity limitations as of 1995. Her income was also adequate throughout, and she continued to live in the same house and drive herself around the community.

Sally had a very diverse pattern of activities that allowed her to adapt very easily. For example, she gradually gave up sports, but she offset this change by increasing her reading and involvement in community organizations. She remained an avid gardener and spent a good bit of time working in her yard. Although she had never married and had no children, she kept in close contact with other family members and had a large network of friends. She attended concerts and lectures very often. She held offices in several community organizations, and in her early retirement years she was elected to local office. She remained very goal directed and active and reported constantly making new friends.

Like Gordon, Sally experienced no life changes that could not be easily accommodated. Even though by 1995 she reported having to rest more often than was the case earlier, she experienced physical, mental, and social aging as a gentle slope, well within her ordinary coping capacity. Also like Gordon, Sally scored very high on our scale of preventive health practices. She also benefited from a strong sense of direction and from a strong personal feeling of spirituality. She also scored high in gerotranscendence.

Lynn and Dennis are a couple who both participated in our study and who also illustrate the pattern of experiencing aging as a gentle slope. Both were in their mid 50s at the beginning of the study and in their mid 70s in 1995. Through the launching of their children and Dennis's retirement, they maintained very positive morale, self-confidence, and expectations or ratings of life in retirement. They also remained active, enjoyed a comfortable level of income, and continued to live in the same home.

Although both remained in good health throughout, both reported that they could no longer do heavy work around the house by 1995. They compensated for this change by hiring help, and their very adequate income allowed them to do so without feeling a financial pinch.

After Dennis retired from his position as a university administrator, his activity level remained high. He offset a decline in participation in professional organizations with increased time spent gardening, volunteering, and working on his hobby of genealogy, for which he had to learn some new computer skills. Dennis remained much in demand as a member of community boards, and in 1995 he continued to serve on several.

Early in the study, Dennis and Lynn were moderately involved in antique collecting, but by 1995 they had ceased this activity completely. They reported that they simply lost interest and increased their time spent in other activities.

Lynn's overall activity level dropped slightly from 1991 to 1995. She exercised less often, spent substantially less time on antique collecting, and she cut back on her involvement in community organizations. Part of this change was offset by her increased involvement in church activities and in the senior center but most was offset by her feeling that she needed more time for ordinary housework, to keep the house up to her own standards. She remained an avid bridge player and shopper.

Lynn and Dennis enjoyed a very happy marriage throughout the study. They enjoyed traveling together, and they enjoyed the additional time together that retirement allowed. They also continued a pattern of having separate activities, which gave them some time apart. Both scored very high on our scale of preventive health practices. Both listed their religious faith, their marriage, their friends, and their family, in that order, as their major means of coping. They shared a common sense of direction, scoring more than 85 percent overlap in their ratings of the importance of various personal goals.

Substantial Change with Positive Outcome

Cynthia experienced significant changes that required substantial adaptation, including having cancer herself and having to be a caregiver for her increasingly chronically ill husband. She came through these changes with a very positive mental outlook and a high overall activity level. Resources that helped her to cope included continued good health, including successful recovery from her cancer, adequate financial resources, a strong network of friends, and a great deal of inner strength.

When our study began, Cynthia was in her early 50s, married, and had two children still living at home. She worked full time as a caseworker for a social services agency. Her husband worked as an accounts manager. She was very satisfied with her marriage. She had above-average self-confidence and average morale, which she maintained throughout the study. Her attitude toward life in retirement was very positive before she retired and remained so. Her overall activity level remained stable and was well above average for the panel throughout the study.

Cynthia herself experience aging as a gentle slope. Physically, mentally, and socially she remained a high-functioning adult throughout. In 1990 she was diagnosed as having cancer, but the treatment was successful as of 1995, and she continued to rate her health as good. She had no physical functional limitations.

But Cynthia's retirement did not turn out as planned. Beginning in 1977, her husband's health began to deteriorate because of a chronic neurological disorder, which forced him to retire earlier than anticipated, and that in turn meant less adequate retirement income than they had anticipated. To compound matters, Cynthia also decided to retire early in order to care for her husband. In 1981 she said, "Our greatest limitation in retirement has been my husband's unpredictable health. This was something we did not anticipate. It's no fun to travel, for example, if you are miserable when you get there."

By 1991, Cynthia and her husband had actually been drawn closer by their need to cope with his health problems. She acknowledged that his condition imposed some significant constraints on her life in retirement, but it also brought them closer and made them "even more mutually supportive." Her overall assessment was that "so far as I am *personally* concerned, retirement is busy, productive, and good. My major concern is about my husband's illness, which is not only restricting but worrisome." Thus, being part of a couple and having a lifestyle that revolved around her marriage meant that her husband's health had a major constraining impact on Cynthia's life. But caregiving had its positive side, too. She felt more needed, and she was gratified by the love and support of family and friends.

How Cynthia adapted her lifestyle to maintain her overall high activity level in the face of significant constraints illustrates the creativity that many aging adults mobilize in the process of coping. Before her husband's illness, Cynthia had a diversified activity pattern that involved gardening, sewing and crafts, collecting, reading, and meeting with small groups of friends who shared her interests. By 1991, she had substantially reduced her involvement with art collecting — they had moved to a small condominium and simply did not have the room — and she was not able to attend social gatherings as often. She had offset these declines by becoming more involved in her church and in community organizations. By 1995, she found herself increasingly tied to the household by her husband's deteriorating condition. She coped with this change by writing prose, poetry, and reflections and posting them on various newsgroups on the Internet. She quickly mastered the computer and the intricacies of the Internet. This creative solution to her need for intellectual stimulation and interaction allowed her to feel less isolated than she otherwise might have. She spent an increasing amount of time on her daily writing and E-mail.

Cynthia coped with the ups and downs of her husband's condition by relying on social support from family and friends, keeping a positive attitude, and by her strong belief in the value of serving others. Although her life has not turned out as she planned, she has creatively fashioned a new close-to-home lifestyle that still allows her to remain engaged with the world outside and to derive great satisfaction from her many interests. In other words, she was able to create a new lifestyle that continued to meet her most important needs, which themselves remained consistent.

Again, planning and intentions were important. Cynthia's good health was related to her high score on preventive health measures. Her positive attitude was related to her understanding of her need for social support and her innovative solutions to continuing to receive social support even as she became more confined to the household. Her creative writing provided an outlet for emotional expression, and her Internet access allowed her to seek information aggressively to manage her husband's illness more effectively. In 1997, Cynthia felt that she was keeping on top of information and meeting her personal needs while doing a good job of caring *with* her husband, which brought her great satisfaction.

Roger was in his mid 50s when our study began. He worked as manager of a retail store and had been happily married for more than 30 years. His overall activity level was about average for the panel, as were his levels of self-confidence and morale. He had a very positive attitude about the prospect of life in retirement, was in very good health, and had a very adequate income.

Roger's plans for life in retirement were substantially disrupted by a stroke that left him almost totally blind in both eyes. In 1991, he reported that he felt very dependent on his wife to help him get around, and his activity level had dropped considerably. His self-confidence and morale also dropped to below average. But by 1995, Roger had successfully adapted to his new situation. He no longer felt dependent on his wife; in fact, he was providing care for her. Feeling needed was important to Roger. He compensated for important lost activities such as reading and spectator sports by increasing his involvement in exercise and in community organizations. As a result, by 1995 Roger's morale and self-confidence were back up to their prior levels, and his rating of life in retirement was even more positive than it had been before his stroke. He felt that perseverance and his strong religious beliefs were the major resources that allowed him to cope.

Joanne was in her early 50s when our study began and in her early 70s in 1995. A never-employed homemaker, Joanne reported herself to be in very good health; her self-confidence, morale, and attitude toward the prospect of life in retirement were all about average for the panel in 1975. Her husband was a university professor, and they had lived in the same house for many years. She reported that her marriage was very satisfactory, and being close to her husband ranked first among her personal goals. Her overall activity level was also about average for the panel. She had an activity profile revolving around socializing — she frequently participated in community organizations and frequently played bridge and got together with friends. She also visited with her children often and spent a lot of time reading.

Joanne's life in retirement did not turn out as she expected because her husband died suddenly in 1989. Although we might expect that a couple-oriented person such as Joanne would be devastated by her husband's death, she eventually adapted to this change quite well. In 1991, she had increased her activity level considerably. Keeping busy was her major coping strategy for dealing with her bereavement. This strategy worked; her morale, self-confidence, and rating of life in retirement all remained at their previous levels. But by 1995, she had settled back into her previous level of activity, and her psychological well-being remained at previous levels.

Joanne credited the community for easing her transition into widowhood. "It's an easy place to live, and that makes adjusting easier." She also felt that keeping her sense of humor and not feeling sorry for herself were also important coping strategies. It also helped that she had a network of friends, some widowed and some still married, with whom she could still be involved in the socializing that formed the core of her previous lifestyle activities. Thus, with a positive attitude, a conducive community, and social support from her friends, Joanne was able to maintain continuity in her life in the face of widowhood.

Unwanted Discontinuity with Negative Outcome

Matilda was in her late 60s and had already retired from her career as a dance teacher when our study began in 1975. She was happily married, in good health, and active. Her self-confidence, morale, and and rating of life in retirement were all well above average. She did not participate in community organizations, but otherwise she had a large and diversified array of enjoyable activities. She had a large network of friends with whom she spent time very often. Her activity level was above average for the panel.

After she retired, Matilda wrote a book on exercises that elders could do to keep limber, and she made the rounds of senior centers in the area presenting programs. This activity was a very important job substitute and source of social recognition for Matilda, who had a high need for ongoing positive feedback about her usefulness to others.

In 1979 she broke her hip, and as a result she was no longer able to present her exercise programs. Her activity level dropped substantially and so did her self-confidence and morale. But by 1981, she had adapted. Her hip had healed, so she was able to get about in the community. She concentrated more on her housewife role and found usefulness in caring for her husband, who was becoming increasingly disabled by chronic heart disease. She also increased her attendance at local senior center activities substantially but this time as a participant rather than as a program presenter. Her activity level was back up and so were her morale and self-confidence.

In 1991, Matilda's health continued to be good. Her activity level had dropped to well below average for the panel, mainly because her husband's condition required giving up travel, being with friends, and attending social gatherings and senior center functions. She offset this somewhat by increasing her church attendance. Her morale and self-confidence remained high, however, because caregiving met her need to feel useful.

By 1995, then in her late 80s, Matilda's situation had changed dramatically for the worse. Her husband had died in 1992. Her own health worsened because her broken hip had not healed properly, which had long-term negative effects on her spine, which in turn limited her mobility even further. Nevertheless, she still rated her overall health as good.

During the time that she was caring for her husband, Matilda became isolated from her friends, and after his death, her own mobility problems made it difficult for her to reengage within the community. In 1993, she moved to a distant state to live with her younger sister and brother-in-law. After more than two years in her new surroundings, she was still very inactive. Her most frequent activities were "eating, sleeping, and dressing." Very little of her 1975 lifestyle remained. In 1995, she never engaged in 14 activities that she had enjoyed in 1975. She reported having no friends.

The results for her psychological well-being are not surprising. Matilda went from having above-average self-confidence, morale, and rating of life in retirement in 1991 to having well below-average scores in 1995. She felt lifeless, useless, dependent, and idle. She felt that her life had not at all turned out as she expected.

These changes far exceeded Matilda's routine coping capacity, and she had little by way of inner or outer resources for dealing with them. Her move to a new community cut her off from social support from her network of friends, which had been somewhat dormant anyway. And Matilda reported few internal coping resources. She had no answer to how she coped with life, perhaps because she had not coped. Having been a frequent church-goer in 1991, she no longer attended. She reported no satisfaction from her inner life and no guiding philosophy of life or sense of direction. She no longer had the self-confidence to make decisions; she reported just letting things happen as they happened.

Being useful to others had been Matilda's single guidepost for the duration of our study, and when circumstances took away her capacity to continue to see herself as useful, she seems to have lost interest in life. Her lack of internal coping resources provided little basis for changing direction late in life.

Wayne was in his early 50s when our study began. He was married with a child still living at home, and he worked as a university professor. His life revolved around his work and family obligations. He was in good health and had average self-confidence and morale. On the other hand, compared with the panel in general, his rating of his prospective life in retirement was much less positive — not negative, just not positive. His activity level was slightly below average. The only activities he reported doing often were engaging in politics, reading, and listening to classical music on the radio.

In 1978, Wayne's wife died, leaving him to care for his teenage daughter who was still living at home. In addition, he developed a heart problem that limited his capacity to do heavy work but otherwise did not affect his lifestyle. He took these changes in stride. He increased the amount of time he spent with his child and took on more household obligations. He cut back on going to sporting events. Otherwise, his life remained a simple one focused on work and family obligations.

In 1983 his daughter left for college and was home only occasionally before moving into her own independent household in a distant city. In 1991, Wayne continued to work, and his health and activity level remained about the same as in 1981. However, his self-confidence and morale suffered from his no longer having family obligations to organize his home life. Nevertheless, he remained satisfied with the amount and use of his free time.

In 1995 Wayne was in his early 70s. He had retired in 1992, and unlike most of our respondents, he had not been very positive about this change beforehand. Before retirement, he had expected his life in retirement to focus on sickness, immobility, incapacity, and dependence. In other words, he thought that poor health would force his retirement. But working conditions had more to do with his decision to retire. He began to feel that the issues that were important within the university community no longer held much interest for him. He experienced less and less empathy for his students and his younger colleagues, less patience with the bureaucracy, and less respect for the university administration. He was befuddled by the compulsory student evaluations of his teaching, which were sometimes unfavorable. These sociocultural factors, more than his health, led him to retire.

After retirement, Wayne felt inactive, uninvolved, and that his life was empty, idle, and meaningless. He had expected sickness, but what he experienced was a crisis of life meaning. Not surprisingly, his self-confidence and morale slipped even further below average. His activity level remained about the same, and he was satisfied with his amount of free time and how he used it. He still focused on reading, listening to classical music, engaging in politics, and playing cards. But Wayne's customary lifestyle had revolved around obligations, not leisure pursuits. He reported that his major means of coping with life was to immerse himself in his obligations to work and family. But by 1995 he no longer had these obligations as coping resources; he no longer worked and had only occasional contact with his daughter. These changes had very negative results for his psychological well-being.

Stella was 60 when our study began. She had a high-school education and was a secretary her entire working life. She never married and had no children, but she had a number of relatives nearby and kept in frequent contact with them as well as with an extensive network of friends. Initially, she reported her physical health as only fair because of chronic asthma, although at that time she could still perform all of the activities on our functional health scale. She had a very diversified pattern of activities, and she engaged in them often. Her overall activity level was well above average for our panel, which was generally very active. Her morale and self-confidence were average for the panel, but she was well above average in terms of her rating of her prospective life in retirement.

From 1975 until 1991, Stella experienced aging as a gentle slope. There were no serious illnesses or life events to disturb the satisfying rhythm of her customary lifestyle. But by 1995 her asthma had become so severe that breathing difficulties had become constant, and substantially decreasing her mobility changed her life considerably. She could no longer walk any significant distance or climb stairs. She began to need assistance from a homemaker service worker. She cut back sharply on her participation in gardening, community organizations, and attending concerts and sporting events. Her increased physical constraints were not ones that can be easily compensated for, and by 1995 she had lost several important elements of her previous lifestyle.

Stella felt that she was sick and uninvolved. Her self-confidence and morale also suffered but still remained in the average range for the panel. Her strong religious faith and strong network of friends allowed her to cope better in terms of psychological well-being compared with the previous two cases. In response to our question "How do you cope?", she said, "Faith in God above all other things, self-determination, and good friends." Stella obviously used both internal and external resources to adjust to her changed circumstances. But the sheer nature of her disability limited her options, and she experienced a sharp discontinuity in her lifestyle, which was obvious in our objective data as well as in her own self-report.

We have seen that continuity and successful adaptation are typical outcomes for aging people. Negative outcomes are rare and are often tied to severe functional limitations. Next, I consider the dynamics associated with negative outcomes in more detail.

Factors Linked to Negative Outcomes in Later Life

In this section I consider the factors related to negative changes such as reduced morale, self-confidence, attitude toward retirement, activity level, self-rated health, and functional capability. I begin with the prevalence of these various negative outcomes.

As I mentioned earlier, a large majority of respondents remained within the positive range of most of our criterion variables throughout the study.

However, a few of our respondents reported negative changes that took them into an absolutely problematic state rather than simply into a relatively deprived state.

For example, the mean morale scale scores for the panel were high, around 33 for all waves of the study. But there were 12 respondents whose morale scores fell from 33 or higher to 27 or lower, which represented a drop of at least 2 standard deviations. Seven respondents reported a substantial drop in self-confidence, from average or above to near the bottom of the positive range of self-confidence. Fifteen respondents reported a dramatic drop from a very positive view of retirement to a neutral or slightly negative attitude. Eleven reported changing from very active to inactive in terms of lifestyle activities. Twelve respondents changed from at least fair self-reported health to poor or very poor, and most dropped from fair to poor. Only one respondent rated his health as very poor in 1995, and no one dropped from very good to poor or very poor among the panel who responded to all six surveys. Finally, 17 respondents who were fully capable in physical functioning at the beginning of the study had developed five or six functional limitations by 1995.

We might expect that these negative changes would cluster together, that negative changes in health and physical functioning would be related to negative changes in the other variables, but for the most part this was not the case. Thirty-seven respondents reported negative changes on only one of the six dimensions listed above; 10 reported two negative changes; 4 reported three negative changes; 1 reported four; and only 1 respondent showed negative changes on all six dimensions.

Negative change in morale was prevalent among those who experienced two or more negative changes. Eleven of the 16 cases showing two or more negative changes involved a negative change in morale. All cases that involved three or more negative changes included negative changes in physical functional capability.

To get a better idea of the dynamics of these negative outcomes, a series of multiple regressions was performed to examine the predictors of low morale, low self-confidence, low rating of life in retirement, and low activity level. Low morale in 1995 was related to a different set of factors for men than for women (see Table 4.19). Among men, low morale in 1995 was related to having lower morale in 1991 and having lower functional capability and self-rated health in 1995. For women, low morale in 1995 was related to having low morale in 1991 and a low 1995 activity level. Thus, for both men and women, continuity of low morale from four years earlier was the strongest

TABLE 4.19. Predictors of morale, self-confidence, life rating, and activity level, 1995

	Dependent Variable				
	Morale		Self-Confidence	Life Rating	Activity Level
Predictor	Male	Female			
Age	−.035	.088	−.046	−.089	−.138**
Gender			.035	.013	.001
Education	−.188	−.116	.026	.119	.009
1991					
Morale	.392**	.514**			
Self-confidence			.351**		
Life rating				.291**	
Activity level					.712**
Friends	.177	.086	.028	.171*	.037
Disposition toward continuity	.002	.114	.456**	.227**	.081
Functional capability	.234*	.143	.092	.074	.016
Self-rated health	.318*	.123	.194**	.354**	.160**
Activity level	.108	.233*	.034	.046	
R^2	.450	.404	.591	.509	.709
N	53	76	162	146	131

* Beta coefficient significant at the .05 level or better.
** Beta coefficient significant at the .01 level or better.

predictor of low morale, but the additional predictors for men related to current health and for women, activity level. The availability of social support (number of friends living in the area), disposition toward continuity, or social structural factors such as age, gender, or education were unrelated to having low morale in 1995. Low morale is not just a response to current health or activity level; the most significant correlate of low morale is low morale in the past. Thus, continuity is an important determinant not only of high morale but of low morale as well.

Low self-confidence in 1995 was predicted by a low disposition toward continuity, low self-confidence in 1991, and low self-rated health (see Table 4.19). There was no gender difference in predictors of low self-confidence. Again, continuity over time is a major force, but here the relationship with continuity reflects not only the persistence of low self-confidence over time but also the low perceived applicability of continuity as an adaptive strategy. Lower self-rated health is also related to lower self-confidence. The R^2 for the model is relatively high (.591). Interestingly, activity level, social support availability, social structural factors, and functional capability were not significant predictors of low self-confidence.

Table 4.19 also shows data for predictors of how respondents rated life in retirement. A low rating of life in retirement is predicted by low self-rated health, low disposition toward continuity, and low availability of friends in the community. There was no gender difference in the set of factors that predicted life rating. The R^2 for the model is high (.501). Activity level, social structural variables, and functional capability were unrelated to life rating.

Taken together, these results dealing with low values of morale, self-confidence, and life rating show that having low scores on these variables in 1995 was not random. Those who were most at risk were those whose morale, self-confidence, and life rating were already relatively low compared with those of the rest of the panel. In addition, those who had low self-confidence and low life rating also did not see themselves as using continuity as an adaptive strategy to the same degree that other respondents did. Not surprisingly, low self-rated health was the other factor that persistently predicted low values on morale, self-confidence, and life rating.

A final regression analysis of predictors of low activity level is also shown in Table 4.19. Having a low activity level in 1995 was related most to having a low activity level in 1991 (beta = .712), followed by low 1995 self-rated health (.160), low 1995 morale (.146), and older age (.138). The R^2 for this model was very high (.709). Like the attitudinal variables analyzed above, low activity level shows a high degree of continuity over time and a relationship to low self-rated health. Unlike the attitudinal variables, low activity level shows a relationship with older age over and above the effects of self-rated health and physical functioning, which were controlled in the regression analysis. Low activity level was not related to a high disposition toward continuity, which suggests that a low activity level is not voluntary or purposeful.

But these regression analyses do not tell the entire story because there are always people who experience the same "predictor" but not the negative change predicted; the R^2 statistics seldom even begin to approach 1.0. Next, I look in detail at specific categories of cases to get a different view of how changes in psychological well-being, lifestyle activities, and health fit together in the lives of people who experience continuity compared with those who experience discontinuity. We are particularly interested in the *sequences* of changes that precede negative outcomes. I look first at cases of continuity.

Among cases showing continuity in outcomes such as morale, self-confidence, life rating, or activity level, 41.7 percent experienced aging as a gentle slope. Their health, psychological well-being, and activity scores remained consistent over the six waves of the study. Another 25 percent experienced a slight decline in self-rated heath, but their psychological well-being scores and activity level remained consistent. The two other patterns involved minimal declines in health, psychological well-being, and activity level (16.7%) and a slight decline in activity level but consistent psychological well-being and self-rated health (16.7%).

The continuity category was noteworthy because continuity was a strong motive among most people in this category. Above-average disposition toward continuity characterized 41.7 percent of these respondents, and another 33.3 percent had an average disposition toward continuity. Only 16.7 percent of the respondents in the continuity category had below-average disposition toward continuity scores. These findings strongly suggest that continuity is an intended outcome. It may be facilitated by having good health or sufficient financial resources, but a key ingredient seems to be the desire for continuity.

The cases of discontinuity provide an informative contrast. Among those who experienced discontinuity, only 11.8 percent were unrelated to declining functional capability. Moving to another community was the factor related to discontinuity in these cases.

In a large majority (70.6%) of cases involving declining morale or activity level, declines in functional capability preceded declines in morale and activity level. This is the conventional wisdom, and it has usually been confirmed in longitudinal studies that have been reported. In another 17.6 percent of cases, declines in functional capability and in psychological well-being and activity level occurred concurrently.

Given the overwhelming relationship between declines in physical functioning and declines in psychological well-being and activity level, it would be easy to presume that the relationship was mainly physical. But surprisingly, 58.8 percent of the discontinuity category scored well below average on disposition toward continuity. What this means, of course, is that a large majority in the discontinuity category reported little motivation to act in ways that would maintain consistency in lifestyles, which, as our case studies showed, was a key element in being able to restore psychological well-being in the face of serious life changes. When we looked at disposition toward continuity among those who were able to restore psychological well-being after disruptive life changes, we found that 67 percent had average dispositions toward continuity, 33 percent had above-average dispositions toward continuity, and none had below-average dispositions toward continuity. In other words, those who successfully restored the balance of their lives after serious life changes were precisely those with motivation to do so.

Summary

Continuity serves the process of adapting to change in two important ways. First, the desire for continuity can motivate people to prepare in advance for changes such as retirement, widowhood, or even disability, all changes that are likely to occur in later life. Second, concepts about both internal and external continuity can serve as a goal for adaptation; that is, faced with serious changes, people often try to preserve as much continuity as possible. Continuity is not just an objective outcome; continuity is also often a highly desired experience.

Most respondents in our study saw themselves as using adaptive strategies built on continuity and aimed at preserving continuity. Most also felt that they had maintained continuity of lifestyle, relationships, and personal values.

Proactive coping involves anticipating and preventing or neutralizing problems. A very high proportion of our longitudinal panel had taken many conscious steps to prevent serious chronic illness and disability, and most of the time these efforts paid off. Most had planned sufficiently to ensure adequate income throughout their retirement.

Reactive coping involves identifying and using coping resources to adapt to challenges. Our panel cited inner factors such as having a positive attitude or religiousness and external factors such as social support and aid from family and friends as coping resources. A high degree of internal and external continuity is often a necessary part of the process of identifying and using coping resources.

When we looked at adaptation to retirement, widowhood, and the onset of functional limitations, we found that continuity played an important role in all types of adaptation. Continuity of lifestyle activities promoted a positive adaptation to retirement, especially for men. Continuity of activities and relationships was also an important coping resource for women who became widowed. Most widowed men remarried, thereby restoring continuity in marital status and living arrangements. Although retirement and widowhood required adaptation, most respondents were able to adapt to these changes successfully.

Adapting to the onset of functional limitations was more problematic. Compared with respondents who retained all physical functions throughout the study, those who developed three or more functional limitations experienced more difficulty maintaining a sense of personal agency, but they were as able as their nondisabled counterparts to maintain their customary level of emotional resilience and goal directedness. The experience of functional limitation did not cause our panel members to revise their basic array of personal goals.

Respondents who had the greatest difficulty preserving their customary lifestyles in the face of disability were those whose functional limitations were caused by systemic conditions such as emphysema, which leave little room for adaptive maneuvering. Panel members who developed less pervasive disabilities were usually able to work around their limitations, offset losses with increases, and preserve a large portion of their customary lifestyles. Most adapted to lost activities by redistributing their energies among remaining ones. Activity disengagement was uncommon and usually connected with severe disability or, in rare cases, by heavy demands of caregiving.

Trajectories of adaptation depend very much on the magnitude of the change that must be assimilated. Most of our respondents experienced aging as a gentle slope punctuated by changes that could be assimilated within a continuity framework relatively easily. A significant minority experienced potentially disruptive negative changes but were able to mobilize coping resources and preserve a significant measure of continuity effectively. A very small proportion of our study participants experienced substantial and disruptive negative changes that were beyond their coping capacity and resulted in long-term discontinuity of viewpoint or lifestyle. But when discontinuity did persist, it was likely to precipitate a loss of morale. Fortunately for our respondents, substantial negative changes did not tend to cluster together.

Those people who had low morale, self-confidence, and life rating in 1995 tended to be people whose morale had all along been relatively low compared with the rest of the panel. They also tended to be people who were not disposed to use continuity as an adaptive strategy. Finally, they tended to be people whose self-rated health was below average when the study began.

5 | Goals for Developmental Direction

As we saw in the previous chapter, aging adults use continuity strategies to anticipate future circumstances and take steps to produce both internal and external continuity. They also use continuity strategies to cope with both routine and potentially disruptive change.

Goals for developmental direction represent vectors of evolution toward which people are oriented and which shape their aspirations and decisions. They are the yardsticks against which the direction of personal change is evaluated. Goals for developmental direction can involve fundamental shifts in perspective toward the self, such as when an individual retires from life as an executive to take up a much less structured life of an artist. But an extreme degree of desired developmental change is relatively rare. Developmental goals that involve continued refinement of personal qualities, skills, knowledge, relationships, or environments are much more common.

In this chapter, I look at several perspectives on goals for developmental direction. First, I consider continuity in personal goals, which, as we saw in Chapter 2, is quite pervasive. Then, I examine disposition or motivation toward continuity as a developmental goal in its own right. I next look at spiritual development as a goal for development that may become more prevalent in later adulthood. I then consider the concept of gerotranscendence as a perspective that may help us understand spiritual development and how it relates to continuity. Finally, I discuss future directions for research on the study of goals for developmental direction in later adulthood.

Continuity of Personal Goals

Continuity of personal goals can be a basis for organizing attention, assimilating change, and making decisions about one's future. Nearly all adults in modern societies are confronted by sensory and conceptual overload. To survive the entropy and chaos of television alone, adults must have a basis for simplifying what they take in. Personal values or goals are used to identify which regions of the environment are important and which can be ignored. Personal goals can also be a framework for assimilating change. For example, Kaufman (1985) found that personal goals were an important tool elders used to interpret change; that is, change was given meaning by its positive, negative, or neutral relationship to personal goals. Finally, as abstract concepts, personal goals provide general guidelines for making everyday decisions about the future, which in turn shape the direction of individual experience; and through feedback, experience shapes individual development.

An inventory of personal goals was part of each wave of data collected in the Ohio Longitudinal Study of Aging and Adaptation (OLSAA). Table 2.9 showed the relative importance of a variety of personal goals. Having close family ties, being dependable and reliable, being self-reliant, being self-accepting, having a comfortable place to live, and being well read and informed were the personal goals that were rated as very important for a majority of respondents who continued to participate in the study. Being prominent in community affairs and being accepted by influential people were rarely considered very important personal goals. Thus, the most important personal goals at the end of our study involved family relationships, personal qualities, and living arrangements. Goals such as having a satisfying job, having a substantial family income, or having roots in the community were very important to only about one quarter of the panel. Goals related to social position in the community were considered unimportant by a majority of the panel.

But how did the respondents' patterns of personal goals change over time? Table 5.1 shows the proportion of respondents by pattern of continuity and change from 1975 to 1995. *Stability* was defined operationally as having the same score over the six waves of data collection. *Consistency* was defined as having a score that fluctuated within the important or unimportant concept space for a particular personal goal. Patterns of discontinuity were classified into those involving a shift from unimportant to important (increased importance) and those involving a shift from important to unimportant (decreased importance). Note that in most cases, patterns of consistency were a more common form of continuity than absolute stability for most goals; being a religious person and doing things for others were the exceptions. Also note that among the top ten personal goals, patterns of discontinuity were uncommon.

More than 90 percent of the 1995 panel respondents showed continuity in their ratings of accepting themselves as they are, being self-reliant, having a comfortable place to live, being dependable and reliable, doing things for

TABLE 5.1. Patterns of personal goals over time (*N* = 302)

Goal	Continuity (%)			Increased Importance (%)	Decreased Importance (%)
	Total	Stable	Consistent		
Accept myself as I am	98.3	44.9	53.4	1.4	0.3
Be self-reliant	97.4	33.9	63.5	1.6	1.0
Have a comfortable place to live	97.4	29.6	67.8	1.9	0.7
Be dependable	97.1	40.6	56.5	2.3	0.6
Do things for others	95.4	48.8	46.6	2.1	2.5
Have close family ties	94.5	42.7	51.8	3.9	1.6
Be well read and informed	90.9	34.6	56.3	5.8	1.3
Have long-lasting friendships	85.4	29.5	55.8	10.1	4.5
Have substantial family income	83.0	28.2	54.8	11.8	5.2
Be a religious person	80.1	45.9	34.2	13.9	6.0
Have close, intimate relationship	71.4	25.2	46.2	16.6	12.0
Be seen as a good person	69.4	20.5	48.9	24.4	6.2
Have roots in the community	68.6	19.9	48.7	19.9	11.4
Seek new experiences	64.2	21.9	42.4	17.9	17.9
Have a satisfying job	59.5	16.2	43.3	10.3	29.6
Be prominent in the community	55.4	21.2	34.2	14.6	30.0
Be accepted by influential people	46.3	18.0	28.3	26.3	27.3

others, having close family ties, and being well read and informed. More than 80 percent showed continuity in their rating of having close long-lasting friendships, having substantial family income, and being a religious person. For a large majority, continuity was within the "important" category. These findings show that personal qualities such as self-acceptance, self-reliance, dependability, serving others, and being well read and informed were rated as important throughout the study by a large majority of respondents. These personal qualities represent personal goals for which progress is largely under the control of the individual. Goals involving maintaining close informal relationships with family and friends were also very likely to be rated as important and to show considerable continuity over the 20-year period. Finally, throughout the study a large majority of respondents thought that comfortable living arrangements and a substantial family income, supporting circumstances for continuity of lifestyles, were important.

On the other hand, goals connected to the larger socioeconomic structure of the community were the most likely to decrease in importance over time. After retirement, about 30 percent of respondents downgraded the importance of having a satisfying job. Being prominent in the community and being accepted by influential people were also likely to be downgraded over time. In addition, the latter two goals were likely to show continuity at the unimportant level; that is, a majority of the panel never thought that being part of the elite of the community was important. These findings support the observation made many years ago by Clark and Anderson (1967) that as they age, people tend to concentrate on personal qualities and relationships and pay less attention to the values that serve the achievement-oriented, competitive world of young and middle-aged adults.

Being seen as a good person by others was the personal quality most likely to increase in importance over time (24.4% of respondents). Seeking new experiences and having roots in the community also showed small but significant proportions of respondents who attached increased importance to them.

The only goal that did not show a majority of respondents with continuity was that of being accepted by influential people. Those who did show continuity were the most likely to feel that this goal was unimportant, but more than half were likely to have changed their rating of this goal, and they were about equally likely to increase the value of this goal (26.3%) as to decrease it (27.3%).

Thus, continuity of personal goals was pervasive within our panel. Most panel members remained highly goal directed in the sense of having a broad array of personal goals they thought were important. Fluctuations over time in ratings of personal goals tended to take place within the "important" category. The enduring personal goals among our panel stressed personal qualities, human relationships, and supports for a comfortable lifestyle.

Disposition toward Continuity

Initial personal goals obviously have a strong impact on subsequent personal goals, but the motivation to produce continuity is higher in some individuals than in others. To examine this dimension in more detail, we developed a

TABLE 5.2. Disposition toward Continuity subscale (N = 303)

	Strongly Agree (%)	Agree (%)	Disagree (%)	Strongly Disagree (%)
When I need to solve problems, I usually try solutions that have worked for me before	11.3	80.7	7.3	0.7
I know myself well enough to know which choices are best for me	14.7	81.6	3.3	0.3[a]
Over the years I have continued activities that suit me and discontinued ones that do not	20.8	75.6	3.3	0.3
My philosophy of life is a consistent force behind the decisions I make	18.1	70.1	10.0	1.7

NOTE: The positive end of the continuum is underlined.
[a] Rows may not add to 100 percent because of rounding.

TABLE 5.3. Disposition toward Continuity, scale distribution

Score	Frequency	Percentage
4.00	1	0.4
8.00	1	0.4
9.00	2	0.7
10.00	8	2.9
11.00	36	13.0
12.00	151	54.5
13.00	27	9.7
14.00	21	7.6
15.00	15	5.4
16.00	15	5.4
Total	277	100.0

NOTE: mean, 12.38; S.D., 1.49.

scale that tapped various dimensions of continuity for the 1995 wave of the OLSAA (see Table 4.1). Factor analysis of the scale revealed that it taps three factors: (1) perceptions of personal agency; (2) perceptions of actual continuity in beliefs, lifestyle, and relationships; and (3) disposition to use continuity strategies. The disposition toward continuity subscale is most relevant for the present discussion. Table 5.2 shows the items and their distribution.

The proportion who agreed with the disposition toward continuity items was extremely high, ranging between 88.6 and 96.3 percent of the respondents. Nearly all respondents had a life philosophy that guided their decision making (abstract personal goals), they had continued activities that suited them and discontinued those that did not (selective investment), knew from experience which activities were good investments, and turned first to time-tested solutions when they needed to solve problems. In fact, such a large proportion of OLSAA respondents endorsed these basic tenets concerning the motivational elements of continuity theory that analyzing the effects of a low disposition toward continuity was difficult — few people were not highly disposed toward continuity.

The scale measuring disposition toward continuity was distributed as shown in Table 5.3. The scale was obviously skewed toward the positive end, with only 17 percent of the respondents falling below the mean. To assess the impact of having a relatively low disposition toward continuity, *t*-tests were used to compare two groups of respondents on the extremes — 47 respondents who scored below the mean (scale score of 11 or lower) and 29 respondents who scored 15 or 16, very high. Because the number of respondents was small, differences between the groups had to be relatively large to be statistically significant. As Table 5.4 shows, those with very high disposition

TABLE 5.4. Activity level, morale, health, and rating of life in retirement, by disposition toward continuity

	Disposition toward Continuity	
	Very High (15,16)	Relatively Low (11 or lower)
Activity level	66.7**	56.0
Morale	33.0*	31.4
Self-rated health	4.2	3.9
Rating of life in retirement	84.3	79.6

* *t*-test significant at the .05 level or better.
** *t*-test significant at the .001 level or better.

toward continuity had significantly higher activity levels and morale compared with those whose disposition toward continuity was below average. However, the two groups were not significantly different in terms of self-rated health or rating of life in retirement, although the direction of differences tended to favor those with high disposition toward continuity. Interestingly, although those with high disposition toward continuity scored higher on perceived continuity in values, friendships, and lifestyles compared with those who scored below the mean, the differences were not great enough to be statistically significant. These findings suggest that perceptions of continuity were tied more to actual continuity of circumstances than to disposition toward continuity.

Why are people motivated toward continuity? First, they see continuity as a foundation for their prospective physical, psychological, and social security. They also see continuity as supporting their purposeful evolution toward their personal goals. Continuity is the maintenance of selective choices they have created over a period of many years; people value predictability, and continuity appears to provide it.

Why are some people not motivated toward continuity? We would expect that people who disliked elements of their past or present circumstances might be less inclined to want to produce continuity. However, having a low disposition toward continuity did not have substantial negative effects, either on objective outcomes such as activity level or on subjective perceptions of continuity.

For most people continuity holds strong attractions, and maintaining continuity and preserving the capacity to use continuity strategies in adapting to change or making life decisions are strong personal goals for developmental direction in their own right.

But individual evolution is not rooted in the past. Instead, it is rooted in the dynamic feedback system that has continuously refined internal and external patterns to serve the individual's needs better. Individual evolution is also rooted in new possibilities for development that occur in later life. Next we turn to spiritual development and wisdom as goals for development that may take on much greater significance in later adulthood.

Spiritual Development

As used here, *spirituality* refers to an inner, experiential domain that can include experiences of organized religion or religious contexts but is not restricted to such experiences. Spiritual experience may occur at many levels: bodily sensations, mental perceptions, emotions, or transcendent states (Atchley 1997a). Spirituality is a quality that can infuse experience in a wide variety of settings. Spiritual experience comes in many forms, ranging from intense experience of the present moment to complete transcendence of the present moment. Spirituality is a holistic inner domain within which individuals deal with existential issues such as the meaning of life, the nature and existence of a greater power in the universe, the causes and cures of human suffering, the meaning of death, and identifying right courses of action.

Spiritual development can be viewed as movement toward ultimate possibilities, and the highest region of spiritual development occurs in the development of a capacity that allows consciousness to transcend the boundaries of body, language, reason, and culture (Alexander et al. 1990; Wilber 1996). Movement toward ultimate possibilities means movement from simple imitative and dependent religious thought and behavior toward a personal cognitive and emotional experience of spiritual issues that integrates both inner and outer life experiences of spirituality; toward subtle, contemplative understanding of the common ground of being that pervades both inner and outer life experiences; toward union with the ground of all being, variously called God, Yahweh, Allah, the Void, the Absolute, or many other names.

Aging does not invariably bring spiritual development, but aging does alter the conditions of life in ways that can heighten awareness of spiritual needs and stimulate spiritual development. Even as a gentle slope, physical aging produces a decline in the body's ability to mobilize physical energy, whereas continuity of mental energy remains a better possibility. Aging usually has little effect on the physical or psychobiological requirements for spiritual awareness. In fact, aging can be something of an advantage. In terms of the capacity to be internally quiet and contemplative, young and even middle-aged people are often hampered by hyperactive lives and excess energy that make them too restless for an inner journey. The moderation of energy levels and biological drives that usually accompanies physical aging can be conducive to patience, meditation, and contemplation.

Psychological aging is accompanied by an accumulation of life experiences with their usual share of paradoxes and contradictions, which in turn reinforce the notion that life is not entirely controllable and certainly not perfectible. Observing the consequences of human behavior over several decades often shows people that most actions or inactions potentially have both positive and negative results. In time, such observations may foster a "let be" attitude toward both the self and others.

Psychologists generally agree that aging is often accompanied by an increase in introspection or reflection (Kogan 1990). Most also see such reflection as an integrative process that usually leads to greater self-acceptance — a view of oneself as a person of worth with both positive and negative attributes (Erikson et al. 1986; Levinson 1990). Indeed, as we saw earlier, self-acceptance was the highest ranking personal goal among the OLSAA respondents. Learning to accept the self holistically with all of its frailties requires rising above personal desires and standards of perfection to a more transcendent viewpoint and learning to witness the personal self without excessively judging are skills that come from contemplative understanding of the self (Epstein 1995).

Numerous observers have noted that adult spiritual development is an incremental process involving mastery of increasingly transcendent aspects of inner life (Alexander et al. 1990; Erikson et al. 1986; Wilber 1996). Achenbaum and Orwoll (1991) tied the development of wisdom to an increasingly transcendent attitude toward oneself, toward relationships with others, and toward worldly aims. Transcendence is a vital dimension of learning to be as one is. Transcending the personal self means focusing conscious awareness on being a simple witness or observer.

The cumulative life experiences that can accompany aging provide an opportunity to develop a base of psychological and social skills from which the individual can exercise the freedom to dwell in inner silence. The burdens of middle age create in most people an "automatic pilot" that can take care of basic needs with only minimal need for intervention and monitoring by the calculative mind. Thus, life experience creates psychological skills and conditions that can promote spiritual development.

Social aging is mostly a process in which society loses interest in the participation of aging people. For example, most Americans complete their childrearing responsibilities by their late 50s, and most retire from employment in their early 60s (Atchley 1997b). Society assigns no new responsibilities to aging people other than to remain self-reliant. Indeed, self-reliance was the second highest-ranking personal goal among our respondents, nearly all of whom were retired. People who have launched their children and who are retired usually have two important advantages in terms of freedom to turn attention to spiritual concerns: a secure income and social permission to focus their attention as they wish.

As age increases, a greater proportion of elders choose a simple household life that revolves around familiar and satisfying relationships, tasks, and activities (Kelly 1993). Most retirees spend significant amounts of time alone, and this alone time can sometimes have a transcendent quality, either in terms of meditative activities or "flow" activities, such as gardening or painting, which, through intense concentration, transport the individual out of the personal self (Larsen et al. 1985; Mannell 1993).

By late middle age, most adults have considerable experience with materialism and social achievement, the conventional prescriptions for personal contentment, and at best find them unpredictable sources of life meaning. Shifts in later adulthood away from acquisition and achievement and toward "secondary goals" such as affiliation and generativity have been documented by a number of investigators (Clark and Anderson 1967; Maehr and Kleiber 1981). Earlier, we saw that goals involving social position tended to be downgraded over time.

By late middle age most adults have also struggled with the loss of meaning that can accompany the deaths of people with whom they had close personal relationships — friends and family members. Dealing with death raises most of the existential issues that form the core of spiritual concerns.

Thus, by late middle age, many people's life experiences stimulate an interest in going beyond the traditional social sources of life meaning to discover more enduring sources. As meaning questions become more salient in later adulthood, the lack of reliable social answers to meaning questions can be a powerful impetus for an inner, experiential quest for meaning. The precise shape such a quest might take often depends on a person's spiritual or religious background. Thus, there tends to be continuity even in the resources used for inner spiritual development.

Although a good logical case can be made that spiritual development represents an increasingly emergent goal for development in later adulthood and old age, studying spiritual development requires concepts, theory, and operational definitions. We next turn to the theory of gerotranscendence as an example of a framework that can be used to assess the extent to which spiritual development is perceived by our respondents as a goal for development that increases in importance with aging.

The Theory of Gerotranscendence

Although the theory of psychological disengagement (Cumming and Henry 1961) has been thoroughly rejected by social gerontology, Tornstam (1994) felt that the rejection of disengagement theory in favor of activity theory was too simple. Tornstam suggested that instead of the *passive psychic withdrawal* of disengagement, elders may instead be showing gerotranscendence, an *involved detachment* from the social and economic agendas that preoccupy young and middle-aged adults. Tornstam felt that the wisdom that can accompany aging can be described best as a shift in metaperspective, in the global conceptions that make up a person's worldview, from a materialistic and rationalistic view toward a more cosmic, transcendent perspective.

Tornstam (1994, 208–9) hypothesized that the shift in metaperspective associated with gerotranscendence was characterized by:

- an increased feeling of cosmic union with the spirit of the universe;
- a redefinition of time, space, and objects away from deterministic, linear conceptions and toward more flexible conceptions of past, present, and future;
- a decreased fear of death;
- an increased sense of blurring of the boundaries between life and death;
- an increased feeling of affinity with past and future generations;
- a decreased interest in superfluous social interaction;
- a decreased interest in material things;
- a decreased self-centeredness; and
- an increased amount of time spent in meditation.

Tornstam's theory is based in part on a presumption that the social conditions and personal objectives of many aging individuals provide an opportunity to slow life down and to experience a mystical union with the divine, however the divine is conceptualized. Once mystical union has been experienced, through nature, prayer, meditation, or whatever, the individual seeking to integrate such experiences into his or her worldview is drawn to the inner sources of mystical union and is less interested in either the egoistic self or various social agendas. From the point of view of the Almighty, what happens to a specific person or social group may become less important.

To evaluate at least some of Tornstam's theory, we used a series of focus groups to refine and revise the gerotranscendence scale initially developed by Tornstam (1994). Our focus group participants had great difficulty relating to Tornstam's ideas concerning altered perceptions of time, space, objects, and the boundary between life and death. Accordingly, this area was omitted from the scale. The final scale consisted of six items and was included in the 1995 wave of the OLSAA. In the initial analysis of the results, the scale reliability was not acceptable (Cronbach's coefficient alpha for the six items was .428). Factor analysis of the six items revealed that the scale was not unidimensional but instead fell into two factors. Table 5.5 shows the items, the distribution of responses, and factor loadings for the two factors: gerotranscendence and present-moment orientation.

The core measure of gerotranscendence appears to revolve around three items: feeling greater connection with the universe, taking more enjoyment from one's inner life, and having less fear of death. These three items form a scale with acceptable reliability (Cronbach's coefficient alpha = .655). Responses to these scale items were in the direction predicted by Tornstam's hypotheses.

The second factor was also made up of three items: "I take myself more seriously," "Material things mean more," and "I feel less connection to past and future generations." Although these items had relatively high factor loadings, they did not form a reliable scale (alpha = .483). In addition, the substantive responses were in the opposite direction from that predicted by Tornstam's theory. For example, 78.4 percent of respondents said that material things meant more, not less, as predicted by the theory. My guess is that material well-being can be taken for granted to a much larger extent in the

TABLE 5.5. Gerotranscendence and present-moment orientation, 1995 (*N* = 294)

Compared with when I was 50	Factor Loading	Strongly Agree (%)	Agree (%)	Disagree (%)	Strongly Disagree (%)
Factor 1: Gerotranscendence[a]					
Death is less frightening.	.646	21.9	60.8	14.6	2.8
I feel greater connection with the universe.	.812	13.0	53.4	27.8	5.8
I take more enjoyment from my inner life.	.804	14.5	64.4	17.8	3.3
Factor 2: Present-moment orientation[b]					
I take myself more seriously.	.713	5.8	48.0	39.5	6.8
Material things mean more.	.765	16.8	61.6	19.2	2.4
I feel less connection to past and future generations.	.622	19.0	49.7	25.2	6.1

[a] Cronbach's alpha reliability coefficient for these three items is .655.
[b] Cronbach's alpha reliability coefficient for these three items is .483.

Scandinavian populations where Tornstam developed his scale. Thus, the respondents in our panel were saying that the material underpinnings of life were more important to them now than when they were 50. However, when we looked at those respondents who had been collectors earlier in our study, we did find evidence of less interest in acquiring new material possessions, which supports Tornstam's theoretical point. This example illustrates very well how important it is to convert abstract, theoretical ideas into crisp operational statements if we are to evaluate theories adequately. Also, contrary to Tornstam's hypotheses, our respondents were more likely to take themselves more seriously, not less, and to see less connection with past and future generations, not more. In interpreting these results, I concluded that transcendence may come in two very different forms. The first is Tornstam's idea of transcendence and does indeed involve growing connection with the universe, interest in one's inner life, and less fear of death. The second involves transcending the past and future to dwell in the present moment, where being present is serious business, material supports are important, and past and future generations are but concepts.

In the literature of spiritual development, there is a longstanding distinction between the transcendent viewpoint of the mindful observer and the transcendent viewpoint of mystical consciousness (Atchley 1997a; Alexander et al. 1990; Wilber 1996). It would seem that the gerotranscendence subscale we developed taps into the transcendent viewpoint of mystical consciousness, but the items in the present-moment subscale, although suggestive, did not do a very good job of tapping the transcendent viewpoint of the mindful observer.

Does gerotranscendence make a difference? Scoring high on the three-item gerotranscendence subscale was highly correlated with being able to maintain morale in the face of disability, independent of other factors that related to maintaining high morale. Thus, developing gerotranscendence in later life appears to be a constructive personal goal that not only increases the capacity for wisdom but can also provide useful detachment from the physical body and its ills. These ideas are suggested by the analysis of our data, but I hasten to add that, promising though it may be, the measurement issues surrounding gerotranscendence theory remain formidable, and much work needs to be done to develop better measures and apply them in a variety of populations.

How does gerotranscendence relate to religion? We might expect that those who think that being a religious person is important would be more interested in spiritual development and might show a greater prevalence of

TABLE 5.6. Gerotranscendence items, by importance of being a religious person (*N* = 294)

	Being a Religious Person		
Gerotranscendence Item	Important	Unimportant	Chi-square
Death seems less frightening (% agree)	85.0	80.9	.209
Greater connection with universe (% agree)	72.5*	59.2	.012
More enjoyment from inner life (% agree)	86.5*	69.6	.023

* Differences significant at the .05 level or better using chi-square.

gerotranscendence. Table 5.6 shows the gerotranscendence subscale item responses by importance attached to being a religious person. Respondents who thought that being a religious person was important were significantly more likely to feel a greater connection with the universe and to take more enjoyment from their inner life compared with those who thought being a religious person was unimportant. However, having less fear of death was not significantly more prevalent among those who were religious.

The Study of Goals for Developmental Direction in Later Life

Numerous investigators have commented on the seeming paradox between the societal negativity about aging in the United States and the extremely prevalent high morale among older Americans. One way to interpret this commonplace finding uses goals for developmental direction as a pivotal theoretical construct. If elders are indeed attracted more to an inner spiritual journey and less to an outer, achievement-oriented agenda, then we could expect that the resulting detachment, which is by definition more self-contained, might well result in higher life satisfaction or morale. This is what we found in our cross-sectional analysis of self-reported change. But retrospective reports are of limited value because the self tends to be a revisionist historian, and longitudinal data are needed to do more definitive analyses of these possibilities.

Continuity can be assessed by an individual in relation to his or her fidelity to a longstanding sense of developmental direction. To the extent that gerotranscendence becomes a developmental goal, it may be an extension of a longstanding spiritual or religious developmental direction. Certainly, we found that most of the characteristics of gerotranscendence were more common among those who valued being religious compared with those who did not. The human mind tends to want concrete, linear answers to questions, but the topic of spiritual development tends to resist logic of this type. To study spiritual development as an emerging goal of development in later life, we must be willing to be much more open to discovery, which in turn means that we need to spend much more time doing exploratory analyses before we will be conceptually ready to move toward highly structured studies.

The theory of everyday mysticism (Atchley 1997a) holds that by freeing older individuals from obligations to the workplace, the family, and the community, society creates conditions under which elders who are so inclined can experience transcendence at least in terms of a present-moment orientation and perhaps even in terms of mystical union with the divine. Outer continuity of lifestyle is often an important support for the inner journey, and most texts dealing with spiritual development acknowledge that a person must have learned the necessary elements of individual and social functioning before he or she will be ready for the liberation that can come with an inner spiritual journey.

There can be little question that having a transcendent perspective on oneself, one's relationships, and one's roles has therapeutic effects in terms of reducing stress and improving physical and mental health (Epstein 1995; Levin 1994). The question is the extent to which elders are able to develop such perspectives on their own or within the context of traditional social institutions. Our preliminary findings suggest that a large proportion of older adults develops a transcendent perspective. What remains is for us to achieve a better understanding of how this development occurs.

A preliminary causal nexus for spiritual development can be sketched out. Young and middle-aged adults suffer from excessive role expectations in terms of productivity and complexity, chronic information overload, and postmodern ambiguities concerning behavioral norms (Klapp 1978). Older adults are much more likely to confront questions of life's meaning than are young adults. Older adults are also much freer to simplify their lives and transcend the hassles of daily living. They can do so quietly and unobtrusively. They need not drop out of community, family, and household life to perform the shift in metaperspective called *gerotranscendence*. Gerotranscendence may involve a balancing in the middle ground between grasping at enlightenment and pushing away the social world. Genuine transcendence may involve being able to resist the urge to grasp or push away. Gerotranscendence serves the important goal of self-acceptance by allowing increased detachment from both the valued and disvalued aspects of the self. If we can observe ourselves as we are in the clear light of pure awareness and resist the urge to praise or condemn, then we may be in a much better position to accept the self in its totality.

6 | Conclusion

Most of the participants in our 20-year longitudinal study of aging and adaptation found aging to be a generally positive experience punctuated by events and challenges that were well within their coping capacity. At the outset, I contended that the high prevalence of aging as a positive experience is not an accident, that it occurs because aging people use concepts of continuity to structure and maintain both mental frameworks and lifestyles, which in turn provides robust resources for coping with even serious and potentially disruptive changes that can accompany aging.

In this final chapter, I go back to the original assumptions and propositions of continuity theory and review the evidence provided by the detailed analyses of data from our longitudinal study. The basic ideas that form continuity theory hold up quite well when reality tested. Next, I look at the issue of whether continuity is an effective coping strategy and if so, under what circumstances. I then review some of the methodological approaches that are a necessary part of using a continuity theory perspective. The chapter ends with some suggestions for future directions in research using continuity theory.

Data used to address the various aspects of this study came from a panel consisting of all persons who were age 50 and older and living in the target Ohio township as of July 1, 1975. This panel was surveyed six times between 1975 and 1995. All panel members were age 70 or older at the time of the 1995 survey. In-depth structured and open-ended interviews were conducted over the course of the study with a small number of respondents who provided much-needed detailed information on individual development and the holistic context within which adaptation takes place. The panel began with 1,274 respondents, but only 335 continued to respond 20 years later. Because we are interested in long-term continuity and adaptation, our analyses focus mainly on those who survived and responded to at least four waves of data collection, including the 1991 and 1995 waves. The panel was primarily white and middle class, but a full range of occupational status and educational attainment was represented.

Assessing Continuity Theory

I begin the assessment of continuity theory with a review of the basic distinctions among stability, continuity, and discontinuity. I then consider how prevalent continuity is across various dimensions of life. Then I look at evidence for the existence of the underlying feedback process that is presumed to create the basic life structure and motivation to maintain it. Next I examine the evidence supporting the basic assumptions and propositions of continuity theory.

Distinguishing Stability, Continuity, and Discontinuity

Change is constant, and many changes can be assimilated into an individual's life without triggering a sense of discontinuity. Stability is a state in which change is imperceptible over time even though change does in fact occur. Continuity is a consistency in *general* patterns of thought, behavior, relationships, and living circumstances over an extended time period. Discontinuity is a relatively serious and potentially disruptive level of change, and adaptation to discontinuity generally requires conscious mobilization of coping resources and efforts to adapt. It is important but difficult to keep in mind that stability is a type of continuity, but continuity allows for much more fluctuation over time in the details of general patterns. In addition, continuity does not mean the absence of change. As a concept, continuity locates evolutionary change in a context that includes the past, present, and anticipated future. Thus, evolutionary links or relationships to longstanding individual patterns are the basis for assessments of continuity and discontinuity, and the kind of continuity that captures people's imagination and harnesses their motivation is much more than a drab or boring sameness. Concepts of continuity are important tools that allow us to blend new experiences into our lives and at the same time be reasonably confident that we will be able to handle the demands such new experiences place on our competence.

How Common Is Continuity?

Table 6.1 shows the prevalence in our panel of continuity and discontinuity for a number of characteristics over the 20-year course of our study. Continuity is a much more common experience than discontinuity for nearly

TABLE 6.1. Prevalence of continuity and discontinuity in the Ohio Longitudinal Study of Aging and Adaptation, 1975 to 1995 (*N* = 309)

Characteristic	Continuity (%)	Discontinuity (%)[a]
Self-confidence	69.3	29.1
Emotional resilience	53.6	44.9
Personal goals	79.2	19.5
Living arrangements	52.4	45.3
Activity level	50.7	47.7
Frequency of interaction		
Family	67.5	30.2
Friends	75.4	23.3
Frequency of participation		
Gardening	56.6	42.7
Community organizations	43.8	56.1
Collecting	58.1	39.6
Reading	83.5	15.2
Perceived continuity		
Lifestyle	54.1	43.3
Friendships	70.5	25.2
Basic values	82.2	12.6
Self-rated health	71.7	27.3

[a] Rows do not add to 100 percent because of missing cases.

all of the dimensions listed in the table. However, the prevalence of continuity is also quite variable across the different general dimensions, ranging from 82.2 percent for perceived continuity of basic values to only 50.7 percent for living arrangements. Thus, continuity is multidimensional and may be high in some areas of a person's life and low in other areas. However, we found that extreme discontinuity was relatively rare and tended to occur only in limited areas of a person's life.

Living arrangements for most respondents were a combination of marital status and duration in the same household. Of those whose marital status changed during the study, 50 percent moved, whereas only 27 percent moved among those whose marital status did not change. Widowhood was a major cause of discontinuity in living arrangements, and this factor was much more likely to affect women than men.

Of the 47.6 percent with discontinuity in activity level, 37.6 percent experienced a substantial decline, and 10 percent experienced a significant increase in activity. Among the 56.1 percent who showed discontinuity in their participation in community organizations, 25.3 percent showed a substantial increase in participation, and 26.9 percent showed a substantial decline. Thus, we should not assume that discontinuity is always undesired or in a negative direction.

Of the 71.7 percent who experienced continuity in self-rated health, 5.6

percent rated their health as only fair, and 66.1 percent consistently rated their health as good or very good. Continuity usually preserves positive patterns, but not always.

If we compare the perceived continuity reported retrospectively by the respondents with the researchers' ratings of continuity based on longitudinal reports, the results match very well. In the area of lifestyle, 54.1 percent of respondents saw themselves as having continuity, and the researchers' assessment reflected 52.4 percent continuity in living arrangements and 50.7 percent continuity in overall activity level. In the area of friendships, 70.5 percent of respondents saw themselves as having continuity, and the researchers' assessment was 75.4 percent continuity in terms of frequency of interaction with friends. In the area of basic values, 82.2 percent of respondents saw themselves as having continuity, and the researchers found that 79.2 percent exhibited continuity of personal goals (see Table 6.1).

Thus, continuity is indeed the prevalent outcome for most of the life dimensions we measured, and both continuity and discontinuity exist in a variety of forms.

Is There a General Model Underlying the Development and Maintenance of Continuity?

Figure 1.1 presented a feedback system model of the continuous evolution of internal and external elements of life structure. We found that most respondents did indeed show a persistent structure of ideas about their self-concept and personal goals as well as consistent patterns of living arrangements, relationships, and activities. Most saw themselves as active and engaged in making important decisions about their lives, and most had used their life experiences to develop ideas about what choices and activities were best for them; they tended to preserve and maintain those choices and activities whenever possible. Thus, the underlying feedback systems model of adaptation was supported by the limited amount of data we could bring to bear on it. However, to test this model more rigorously requires much more specific longitudinal data on many more feedback loops than we were able to include in our study. I return to this issue later in the discussion of future research.

Evidence on the Assumptions and Propositions of Continuity Theory

In this section, I examine the various assumptions and propositions one by one to see how well they stood the test of our longitudinal data.

Assumptions

Continuity means evolutionary consistency and linkage over time; stability or equilibrium is a type of continuity, but evolutionary forms of continuity are more common. To arrive at estimates of objective continuity that closely matched the respondents' assessments, we had to use a more inclusive definition of continuity rather than the more limited definition offered by absolute stability. This implies that the respondents saw continuity as a general concept, not a concept tied closely to intricate details of daily life. With a few exceptions, continuity that allowed for limited fluctuation over time was much more common than stability.

Continuity over time is observed commonly in the psychological, behavioral, and social patterns of aging individuals. In Chapters 2 and 3, we found over and over again that continuity was a very prevalent pattern. However, we also found that continuity was most prevalent in general frameworks of ideas, followed by continuity in social interaction. Continuity of activities was much more variable, and continuity in overall activity level was often achieved by offsetting increases and decreases in specific activities. Nevertheless, one of our findings was that respondents tended to persist with the basic pattern of activities they showed at the beginning of our study.

In our time-lagged regression analyses, continuity over time in the dependent variable was invariably the most important predictor. This is another important type of evidence for the power of the continuity principle.

Continuity usually coexists with discontinuity. Virtually everyone in our study experienced discontinuity. For example, nearly all retired from employment and went through the retirement transition. Many launched their children into adulthood during our study. Some experienced life-threatening illness and some the onset of functional disability. But for most of our respondents, continuity far outweighed discontinuity.

Continuity is more evident in general patterns than in the specifics subsumed under general patterns. Regardless of the dimension, we found across the board that there was much more fluctuation over time in specific activities or attitude items than in overall scale scores.

Individual perceptions of reality consist of personal constructs that individuals actively develop by learning from life experience. Internal and external patterns of continuity are highly individuated. Culture and socialization influence personal constructs but do not determine them.

Whether we consider mental constructs of personal agency, the structure of personal goals, or individual activity patterns, each individual in our study was truly unique, and no two data profiles were identical even though we used many standardized measures. For many of the constructs we studied, there were dozens of different patterns of continuity. Respondents often planned in advance to follow the cultural norms regarding the timing of life course events, but many adapted their actual behavior to take personal considerations into account, and few expressed any hesitation in doing so. Of course, American culture stresses individualism, so this should not be surprising.

Individual patterns of adaptive thought continue to develop throughout life. The creativity our respondents used to maintain continuity was inspiring. Recall the case of Cynthia, who reconciled her need to be at home to care for her frail husband and her need for human interaction by using the Internet as a source of interpersonal exchange. Roger learned how to resume golfing even though he had become blind. These are dramatic cases, but I was impressed with the large number of respondents in our study who were always on the lookout for ways to protect and preserve their customary way of life, not out of fear or defensiveness or rigidity but because their customary way of life was a rich source of potential life satisfaction for them.

Using continuity strategies to pursue goals or adapt to change does not necessarily lead to successful results. "Successful" aging is in the eye of the beholder, and for most it is highly subjective. People whose adaptation had never been very good still attempted to preserve their customary patterns, often with unsatisfying results. Recall Wayne, who was still trying to structure his life around job and family responsibilities long after he no longer had these responsibilities. Clinging to his past model of adaptation did not serve Wayne well, and his morale plummeted.

Propositions

General patterns of thought, behavior, and relationships are robust and can accommodate considerable change in detailed patterns without triggering a sense of discontinuity. We found that general constructs such as self-confidence, emotional resilience, personal goals, rating of life in retirement, overall activity level, functional capability, and self-rated health remained consistent over the course of the study for a large proportion of respondents, especially in the absence of functional limitation. Less profound changes such as retirement and widowhood tended to have little effect on these general constructs.

Many of our panel respondents who showed continuity in their overall internal frameworks of ideas and external lifestyles nevertheless experienced frequent fluctuations, which most often took the form of offsetting increases or decreases in the degree to which they agreed with various ideas or participated in various activities. We also found that as long as respondents could preserve the pattern of their customary activities, they could experience a decline in overall activity level without feeling a sense of discontinuity in their lifestyle.

Through decision making about self-concept, life course, and lifestyle and experiencing the consequences, individuals acquire a sense of personal agency. Our respondents very definitely had a sense of personal agency. A very large proportion (78.6%) of our respondents saw themselves as active decision makers, not just passive reactors to life circumstances. And they saw their decision making as being effective; 87.5 percent felt that their choices turned out as well as they expected.

Most of our respondents had already developed robust self-concepts and enduring lifestyles by the time our study began, when all were in their 50s or older. However, we did encounter cases in which life course events stimulated adaptation, which in turn increased the respondent's sense of personal agency. Recall the case of Roger, whose self-confidence was shattered by his becoming blind. But the experience of adapting to his blindness successfully and being able to care for his wife brought his self-confidence back to a very high level. Also recall the case of Giles, for whom coping with his own chronic illness and caregiving for his wife were accompanied by a significant increase in his sense of personal agency.

Enduring patterns of thought, behavior, and relationships are the result of selective investments of time and attention made by individuals over a period of many years. People are motivated to protect those investments.

Almost all (96.3%) of our panel agreed that "over the years, I have continued activities that suit me and discontinued ones that do not." Our panel also overwhelmingly (96.3%) agreed that "I know myself well enough to know which choices are best for me." Thus, our respondents very definitely saw themselves as having the knowledge needed to make selective investments of time and energy and as having done so over an extended period of time.

When we looked at lifestyle activities, we saw a great deal of individuation in the patterns that people maintained over the course of our study. And when our respondents were confronted with challenges such as the onset of functional limitations, they usually tried to restore their customary pattern of activities to the greatest extent possible. This indicates that they valued protecting the investments they had made in activity skills and relationships.

Continuity of general patterns of thought, behavior, and relationships is the first strategy people usually attempt to use to achieve their goals and adapt to changing circumstances. A large proportion (78.6%) of our panel agreed that "when I need to solve problems, I usually try solutions that have worked for me in the past." When we looked at how people adapted to the onset of disability, we found that the most frequent response was to use their structure of activities as the basis for adaptation. Aging people in general react to role loss by redistributing their energies to the structure of roles that remain. Which roles they choose to receive increased attention and energy is a highly individual matter, as continuity theory leads us to expect. A common pattern of response to the onset of functional limitations was to preserve the basic pattern of customary activities but at a lower level of participation. Indeed, as long as respondents were able to preserve at least some of their customary activities, they seem to have been protected from feelings of disengagement and loss of morale in connection with the loss of physical functional capabilities. Thus, continuity was an extremely important resource for coping with discontinuity.

Continuity of personal goals provides people with an enduring sense of developmental direction. Personal goals are abstract, idealized conceptions that are seldom achieved completely. As such, they represent enduring guideposts for motivation and decision making. As we saw in Chapter 5, continuity of personal goals is quite high indeed, with more than 80 percent of the panel showing continuity in the degree of importance they attached to most of the goals in our personal goals inventory.

In addition to the personal goals in our inventory, we also looked at the extent to which spiritual development and gerotranscendence assume greater importance as goals for developmental direction in later life. Most of our respondents (78.9%) felt that their inner life had become more important to them compared with when they were 50; and 66.4 percent felt a greater connection with the entire universe. This development inward was associated with lessened fear of death. Thus, long-standing personal goals remain important sources of guidance, but goals for an inner journey of spiritual development came to the forefront for a great many of our respondents as they moved further into later life.

| | | | | |

In general, findings from the Ohio Longitudinal Study of Aging and Adaptation (OLSAA) strongly support the basic assumptions and propositions of continuity theory. The findings reinforce the idea that continuity is multidimensional and that some patterns are more likely to show continuity than others. The findings also support the idea that continuity does not occur by inertia or chance. Continuity was recognized as an intentional decision-making and adaptive strategy by a large proportion of our panel.

Continuity Strategies Are Generally Effective

If we judge the effectiveness of decision making by the results for life satisfaction, then our findings show that continuity strategies are generally effective. Our panel had developed customary frameworks of ideas and patterns of activities and relationships by the time our study began, and they attempted to preserve these structures over the course of our study. Those who were able to do so also experienced continuity of life satisfaction. Those who were able to restore some semblance of internal and external continuity after substantial and potentially disruptive change also tended to restore their morale to its customary level. In addition, those who experience desired and positive discontinuity were moving in a desired direction and tended to maintain high morale. But those who experienced unwanted negative discontinuity in attitudes and lifestyle were very also likely to experience negative discontinuity in self-confidence and morale.

Nevertheless, continuity is not a magic prescription for "successful" aging. For example, among people who have invested themselves heavily in job and family roles to the exclusion of other sources of life satisfaction, attempting to preserve continuity by clinging to the past is not a practical resource for making decisions about the future that are likely to provide continued life satisfaction. Likewise, people who ignore their functional limitations and retain unrealistic expectations of continuity are likely to be unhappy with the results.

Methodological Issues Related to the Study of Continuity Theory

Continuity theory has been discounted on the grounds that it is too general to be tested. It is true that continuity theory does not provide a recipe for successful aging, nor does it describe a dominant pathway for adaptation to aging. However, continuity theory does provide a conceptual framework that can be used to identify general mental constructs and general patterns of activities and relationships and to differentiate continuity from discontinuity operationally over time. It contains a set of assumptions and propositions that can be tested operationally, provided that the investigators have longitudinal data. This book contains numerous examples of how to define continuity operationally using a variety of types of measures and analytical techniques.

The blending of quantitative and qualitative analysis is also an important requirement for assessing continuity theory adequately. Quantitative analysis is very useful in establishing the proportions who exhibit various patterns over time and in sorting out the relative influence of various causal factors. However, because continuity theory is rooted in individual life histories, qualitative analysis is required to understand complex interrelationships over multiple waves of data collection spanning long time periods.

Many of the frustrations researchers have experienced in trying to use continuity theory stemmed from trying to use continuity theory with cross-sectional data. Without data on the same individuals over an extended time period, continuity theory indeed cannot be tested because continuity theory is designed to explain long-term evolution in general frameworks of ideas and patterns of activities and relationships.

Finally, in analysis of longitudinal data, including baseline values for dependent variables in regression analysis is vital. Because continuity over time in the dependent variable is usually a powerful predictor, omitting baseline values for the dependent variable usually overstates greatly the relative usefulness of other independent variables and underestimates the true extent to which the dependent variable can be predicted from knowledge of prior circumstances.

Future Research Using Continuity Theory

Although this book provides a great deal of supporting evidence for continuity theory and shows how continuity theory can be used in longitudinal research, the evidence is limited in generalizability. First, the panel population was certainly representative of the target community, but it in no way represents the diversity of the national population, much less the populations of other parts of the world. For example, continuity strategies are probably more feasible in small towns like the target community than in the relatively anonymous suburbs of large metropolitan areas, where a sense of community is often lacking. In addition, continuity theory probably fits individualistic cultures that emphasize self-determination better than it does cultures that emphasize conformity to collective norms. Continuity theory may well apply better to planners than to people with more fatalistic worldviews, and some cultures encourage planning more than others. This is just a sampling of considerations that make it important to study continuity in a variety of populations and a variety of cultures.

Any single study is always limited in terms of the number of mental constructs and lifestyle dimensions that can be included. Although the OLSAA contained a large number of measures that had direct application to continuity theory, the quality of measures can always be improved, and the number of constructs can always be increased. For example, the OLSAA contained little information on personality and temperament, two very important internal constructs. Continuity theory might prove to be a useful framework for analyzing long-term panel data on personality and temperament. Our measures of personal goals and activity profiles were generally inclusive, but a larger number of goals or activity types would improve the capacity to identify individual structures.

Our study did not include data that directly addressed the use of feedback to modify personal constructs. This would require a very different type of study, one that looked at the process of decision making, interpretation of results, integration of results into mental and lifestyle constructs, and the extent to which feedback was recurrent and had long-lasting results. Such a study would focus on a very different part of the process of creating continuity, a part that was well beyond the design and scope of the present study.

Another frustration that investigators have experienced in trying to use continuity theory stems from the fact that the term *continuity* has two somewhat conflicting meanings in the English language. The most common colloquial meaning of *continuity* implies no change, which is not the meaning upon which continuity theory is based. Instead, continuity theory is based on an evolutionary concept of continuity as recurring themes and persistent patterns in which details can change as long as basic patterns are maintained. The literary concept of continuity captures the idea well. *Continuity of character* does not mean that nothing happens to a character in the story but rather that the character remains recognizably unique over time. This is an evolutionary concept of continuity. Many researchers start out with a flexible, evolutionary definition of continuity in their preamble only to revert to the "no change" definition when they define continuity operationally. I hope that the methods presented in this book showing how to define continuity operationally and with flexibility can help future researchers retain a focus on an evolutionary concept of continuity. Static definitions of continuity do not reflect the meaning of it to our respondents, nor do they meet the basic assumptions of continuity theory.

Of the themes raised in this book, the idea that spiritual development becomes a higher-priority personal goal in later life needs the most work. Although the theory of gerotranscendence makes a good beginning toward explaining why this may occur, the theory needs further conceptual refinement. In addition, we are still struggling to find meaningful language that can be used to collect data in this area. For example, concepts such as religion, spirituality, transcendence, and mysticism are far from achieving agreed-upon definitions even among scholars, and the general public is often very confused concerning what these various terms mean. Because spirituality is an inner realm, personal construct methods may be an important way to discover the language, concepts, and meanings people use to map the territory of their inner landscape that we researchers call spirituality. In any case, much work needs to be done before we can be confident about the extent to which spiritual development becomes a more important personal goal in later life and the effects that this shift may have on decision making and adaptation.

In all of my work thus far, continuity theory has been applied to individuals. But feedback systems theory is equally applicable to groups, and continuity theory could be adapted easily and used as a framework for studying families, peer groups, or organizations. For example, instead of focusing on personal constructs and individual idea frameworks and patterns of activities and relationships, studies using continuity theory to understand continuity and discontinuity in families might focus on socially constructed family culture as consisting of multiple frameworks of ideas, patterns of family activities, and patterns of family relationships. Like individuals, families make decisions and use coping resources to adapt to change. Families often have goals for developmental direction, often involving increased education for the young or accumulating greater material resources. Certainly maintaining continuity of family ties is an important issue for most families. Similar modifications could be used to apply continuity theory to peer groups or organizations. However, it is important to remember that longitudinal data would be needed to apply continuity theory in these contexts too.

| | | | |

I believe that this book illustrates amply the promise of continuity theory as an explanatory framework that can be used to understand how a large majority of aging individuals manages to experience aging as a gentle slope and as a positive experience, despite the modestly negative effects of aging on physical and mental functioning and despite the widespread erroneous beliefs in our culture about the extent and degree of negative effects of aging and the high prevalence of age discrimination in our social institutions. One reason aging individuals may place greater focus on spiritual development is that it is a functional area in which continuity and growth are possible in the face of substantial negative change in physical and mental functioning. For example, research on cognitive functioning shows that age decrements are confined mainly to psychobiological functions and are much less likely to occur in "higher" mental processes such as integration. This is why a greater proportion of elders has been found to exhibit the quality we call *wisdom* compared with young or middle-aged adults.

Most aging adults use continuity to create and maintain a personal system that provides direction and life satisfaction and that does not depend heavily on what strangers think about the effects of aging or what social institutions offer in terms of opportunities for continued participation. This is not to say that ageism and age discrimination do not matter. They very much constrain the field within which most people can anticipate future continuity, and the patterns of continuity people use in later life today might be very different if ageism and age discrimination did not exist.

Tables

TABLE A.1. Mean emotional resilience, by survey wave, for the total panel and 1995 respondents

	Total Panel			1995 Respondents		
Year	N	Mean	S.D.	N	Mean	S.D.
1975	867	26.02	3.6	270	26.78	3.0
1977	701	25.25	3.9	270	26.25	3.7
1979	583	25.50	3.9	270	26.61	3.5
1981	570	26.21	3.7	270	27.17	3.4
1991	387	25.88	4.0	270	26.48	3.7
1995	270	25.66	3.9	270	25.66	3.9

TABLE A.2. Selected predictors of emotional resilience, 1995 ($N = 196$)

Predictor	Standardized Beta Coefficient
Age	.058
Gender	.043
Education	.028
1995	
Health	.197*
Functioning	.009
Activity	.145*
1991 Emotional resilience	.550*
Adjusted R^2	.503

* Beta coefficient significant at the .01 level or better.

TABLE A.3. Mean personal goals scores, by survey wave, for the total panel and for 1995 respondents

Year	Total Panel			1995 Respondents		
	N	Mean	S.D.	N	Mean	S.D.
1975	796	28.09	5.3	224	28.12	5.0
1977	739	27.60	5.3	224	27.60	5.2
1979	590	28.04	4.9	224	28.13	4.9
1981	588	28.17	5.3	224	27.91	4.7
1991	325	28.77	4.9	224	28.61	4.7
1995	224	28.82	4.9	224	28.82	4.9

TABLE A.4. Mean negative beliefs about retirement scores, for the total panel and for 1995 respondents

Year	Total Panel			1995 Respondents		
	N	Mean	S.D.	N	Mean	S.D.
1977	710	18.98	4.5	282	19.06	4.1
1979	651	19.56	4.4	282	19.46	3.7
1981	643	18.90	4.2	282	18.76	3.7
1991	389	17.84	4.0	282	17.90	4.0
1995	284	17.60	3.8	282	17.60	3.8

The Ohio Longitudinal Study of Aging and Adaptation

Principal Investigator: Robert C. Atchley, Ph.D., Scripps Gerontology Center, Miami University

History

The Ohio Longitudinal Study of Aging and Adaptation (OLSAA) research proposal was submitted to the National Institute of Mental Health in June 1973. It proposed a community-based ten-year longitudinal panel study of the impact of retirement on individual social and psychological adjustment and on the prevalence of symptoms of aging, specifically poor health and physical disability. The project received a positive review and was approved for a five-year period that began in January 1975. Funding for the project during the first five years emphasized data collection because time would be required for sufficient retirements to occur in this naturalistic study. The NIMH continued to fund the project until 1982. From 1990 through 1997, funding came from the Ohio Long-Term Care Research Project and the Scripps Gerontology Center. Data were collected in 1975, 1977, 1979, 1981, 1991, and 1995. Thus, the project generated data spanning a 20-year period. Procedures and results are detailed below.

At the time the OLSAA was proposed, few retirement studies had included both genders, allowed retirement to be examined in a longitudinal panel context, took community opportunity structures into account, surveyed people on the margins of the labor force, included spouses of older workers, and collected a large array of social psychological data.

Data collected by this project have been archived at Duke University and Radcliffe College, as well as at Miami University, and numerous investigators have used these data to write theses, dissertations, book chapters, and journal articles. To date, project research reports have focused on such topics as the process of retirement, gender differences in the retirement experience, adjustment to widowhood, the impact of retirement on couples, attitudes toward retirement, activities in middle age and later life, predictors of morale, values of husbands and wives in retirement, the impact of retirement on leisure participation, and the impact of disability. The OLSAA represents a rich source of data for studying the relationships among life events, physical and economic changes associated with aging, life stages, life structure, and psychological and social adjustment.

Purpose

The study had several goals that revolved around testing theories about the effects of retirement. In the early 1970s, retirement was still portrayed in the gerontology literature as a traumatic event, one that caused ill health, mental depression, and social isolation. At that time carefully done research reports were emerging which showed that negative responses to retirement were in the minority (Streib and Schneider 1971; Atchley 1971a, 1971b, 1974).

Atchley (1975b, 1976c) developed two theories that attempted to explain the types of circumstances under which retirement might lead to adjustment challenges. The first predicted sets of circumstances that could be expected to result in role replacement, role consolidation, or role disengagement as a response to retirement. The second was based on the notion of phases of retirement, and it predicted that negative effects of retirement would be associated with a disenchantment phase. Accordingly, the study was designed to collect data to assess these theories. The goal was to identify circumstances under which retirement caused individuals to readjust their ideas and life-styles significantly. In particular, stressful phases of retirement were to be identified and evaluated in terms of their effects on social and psychological adaptation.

A second objective was to look at the impact of retirement and aging on adaptation, defined primarily in terms of physical functioning and morale. This goal was designed particularly to test the continuing assumption in the popular culture that retirement had negative effects on physical and mental health.

A third objective was to examine the relative importance of retirement compared with other life changes such as widowhood, income decline, and physical decline, which could be expected to influence social and psychological adaptation. Many early studies looked at retirement in isolation and attributed changes to retirement that could have been caused by other factors. This study was designed to place retirement in a competing-causes framework that would allow its relative weight as a source of adjustment problems to be assessed compared with other factors such as widowhood or the onset of limitations in physical activity.

A longitudinal panel design was proposed to facilitate identifying phases of retirement and linking them to psychological and social adaptation. To assess individual change, it is necessary to follow the same individuals over time. Measures before and after retirement were particularly important to establish causal order for retirement as well as other changes.

When the initial three waves of data collection showed very positive levels of physical, social, and psychological functioning regardless of employment/ retirement status, the goal of explaining negative responses to retirement could not be achieved. There simply were too few people who had negative experiences associated with retirement. Accordingly, the focus of the study was shifted away from retirement toward physical disability, which in the data analyses had shown far more potential than retirement for being a predictor of adjustment problems such as declining activity levels, morale, or self-confidence. Eventually the study collected data using several different measures of physical functioning. When it became clear that life in retirement was punctuated by caregiving episodes for many respondents, items on caregiving and receiving were included from the 1981 survey on.

Although initially designed to study retirement, the study included measures for several other potential causes of adjustment problems: activity or role loss, launching children into adulthood (the empty nest), widowhood, residential mobility, income declines, health declines, and the onset and severity of disability. This flexible quality meant that the study could be refocused on other issues when retirement turned out not to produce important health or adjustment effects, which in itself was a worthwhile finding (Atchley 1982b).

The OLSAA data files represent a rich array of high-quality panel data collected from a representative community population and spanning a period of 20 years.

The Community

Earlier studies of retirement had a variety of sampling problems. Some used occupational and work establishment samples (Streib and Schneider 1971; Friedmann and Havighurst 1954; Simpson and McKinney 1966; Pollman 1971) that seriously underrepresented workers at the lower end of the occupational status structure. Others (Fillenbaum 1971) were based on samples from health insurance organizations, which again underrepresented people of lower socioeconomic status. Early national longitudinal sample surveys of employment and retirement such as the National Longitudinal Survey of the Labor Market Experience of Men surveyed only men; included very limited health, activity, or social psychological data; and focused mainly on job history and financial data (Parnes 1981). Analysis of data from the Social Security Administration consisted mainly of the demographic characteristics of retirees (Palmore 1964).

The OLSAA was begun as a community-based study. In theory-testing studies, replicating national proportions is less important than having a range of people who experience the processes that are to be explained. Much of the context within which retirement and aging take place depends on the nature of the local community, a variable extremely difficult to capture in national representative samples. Focusing the study on a single community held constant the opportunity structure for participation in various aspects of everyday life. Thus, observed individual differences in such factors as leisure activities or social participation are not confounded by unmeasured differences in community opportunity structures.

The OLSAA was conducted in a small-town Ohio community with a population of about 25,000. The town is rich in opportunities for participation in a wide variety of leisure activities and voluntary organizations and also in amenities such as health care facilities and services, higher education, recreational facilities, and cultural events. The town is on the fringe of a major metropolitan area, but it is distant enough from larger cities that it remained relatively free of major urban problems such as violent crime, urban decay, traffic congestion, and air pollution throughout the study period.

The economic base of the town includes a medium-sized university, several modest-sized factories, a general hospital, a large number of retail establishments and restaurants serving a rural region, several building construction firms, a modest public works department, and many providers of maintenance and repair services. A picturesque central part of the town contains a variety of shops that cater particularly to the college students, their visiting family members, and tourists from a nearby state park, whereas relatively new discount shopping areas and fast-food strips line the outskirts. The town has an atmosphere of economic vitality.

Politically, the town is very diverse and only mildly skewed toward the conservative end of political opinion on many issues, especially compared with with the surrounding county, which is very conservative. The town has an active council/city manager form of government with vocal citizen involvement on almost every type of decision. Socially, there are more than a dozen large churches and several large voluntary organizations that sponsor a substantial number of community service programs in which older residents play important roles both as service providers and as clients. The town has an excellent public library that makes extensive use of older volunteers. It has a spacious, attractive senior center that operates a bus transportation service for elders in the community. The community offers a basic array of Older Americans Act–funded services, including home-delivered meals and home-based personal care.

Small college towns have become a major destination for retirement migration because middle-class people see them as optimal areas in which to live. The presence of the students provides a boost to the economic base, allowing a level of services and facilities that would not be feasible with just the nonstudent population. The students bring an air of vitality and energy with them, and they create a multigenerational atmosphere in what otherwise would be a relatively old community in terms of population age. The university offers an array of concerts, plays, museums, sporting events, and lectures that the elders in the community patronize widely. The presence of the students also provides the critical mass needed for first-class professional services, including physical and mental health care, education, legal services, social services, and financial services.

In population structure, culture, social structure, and economic structure, the town selected for this study is typical of dozens of small college towns throughout the Great Lakes region of the United States.

The Study Population

Based on the U.S. Census data for 1970 and 1980, the population of the township age 50 and older was about 1,805 in 1975. Our goal was to identify every adult in the township who would be age 50 or older as of July 1, 1975, and to survey them all. Thus, the plan was to study the entire population rather than a sample.

Four sources were used to identify prospective study participants:

— voter registration records, which included birth date;
— welfare records, which included age;
— a postcard census of all mailing addresses in the area requesting names and ages of all people in the household who would be 50 or older as of July 1; and

—a review of the telephone directory by several long-time community residents who served as informants.

Names, ages, and addresses collected by these various methods were merged into a single population record consisting of 1,858 prospects. This file overestimated the actual population of eligible panel members because the names generated by the various sources did not always correspond. For example, the same person might be listed in the voter registration records as Eva Maitland Symes, in the postcard census as Lanny Symes, and in the telephone directory as Mrs. Charles Symes. Because there was no cost-effective way to eliminate these duplications, we sent surveys to all ambiguous prospects. As a result, we could only estimate the response rates to our survey based on the intercensal midpoint of the population of the township, which was 1,805 people age 50 and older in 1975. A total of 1,271 people responded to at least one wave of the study, which represented 70.5 percent of the estimated target population.

Research Design

The OLSAA was designed as a biannual survey. The plan was to survey the target population in 1975, 1977, 1979, 1981, 1983, and 1985. However, as a result of funding cuts, the 1983 and 1985 resurveys could not be conducted. Refunding allowed resurveys in 1991 and 1995.

Data were to be collected primarily by mail, with telephone follow-up and interviews for a small proportion of potential respondents, mainly the visually impaired, who were unable to complete the mail questionnaire. The cognitively impaired were to be excluded from the study because they would be unable to respond effectively to the survey questions. Thus, the study design intentionally underrepresented cognitively impaired people.

Historically, mail surveys had a poor reputation in the research methods literature because it was presumed that they yielded low response rates and could only include superficial questions (Selltiz et al. 1962). However, as more research has been done using mail surveys, it has been discovered that well-administered mail surveys are in many ways equal to interview surveys and very much more cost effective. Based on experience with the mail survey format of the 1970 U.S. Census, it was clear that reasonably sophisticated surveys could be conducted successfully by mail. In addition, mail surveys of middle-aged and older samples by the Scripps Gerontology Center had routinely generated response rates greater than 80 percent (Atchley 1969, 1971a, 1971c; Seltzer and Atchley 1971; Atchley and George 1973).

Particularly in surveys that use close-ended response formats, mail surveys are comparable to interviews in terms of response rates and data quality. They also have the advantage of being subject to less social desirability bias compared with face-to-face interviews. Apparently there is less pressure to give socially desirable responses on a piece of paper than in an interview.

Concepts, Measures, and Questionnaire Construction

The data collected in each wave were designed to address several conceptual categories of data:

— demographic data, such as age (date of birth), gender, race, religious preference, household composition, residential mobility, and duration of residence at current address;

— social status characteristics, such as educational attainment and occupational status, as measured by the scale used by the U.S. Bureau of the Census;

— employment/retirement data, such as occupation, most recent job title, hours and weeks worked; employment/retirement status, job skills, exposure to mandatory retirement rules, retirement age or planned retirement age, length of time retired; and spouse's retirement status and spouse's retirement age or planned retirement age;

— economic information, such as income, income adequacy, pension eligibility and pension receipt, by pension type, and perceived income needs;

— relationship characteristics, such as marital status, duration of marriage; number, gender, and ages of children; number of children and close friends living in the immediate geographic area; and effect or expected effect of retirement on marriage;

— health and physical functioning data, such as overall health rating, perceived health trend, functional capability; degree of activity limitation, specific activities limited, and cause of limitation; Activities of Daily Living (ADL) and Instrumental Activities of Daily Living (IADL);

— caregiving experience, either as caregiver, care recipient, or both;

— social psychological data, such as mental rigidity, attitudes toward work, degree to which job goals were met, attitudes toward retirement, beliefs about the effects of retirement, anxiety level, satisfaction with use of time, satisfaction with activities, personal values or goals, morale, self-confidence, and marital satisfaction;

— social participation data, such as types and number of activities and frequency of participation, unmet activity needs, activity level, most highly valued activities, and participation in community organizations;

— other data, such as primary mode of transportation and provision of financial or social support to others outside the household.

In selecting measures for this large array of concepts, existing close-ended scales designed or validated for use with aging and older respondents were given first priority to generate data that could be compared directly with results from other studies. For example, attitude toward retirement was assessed using a 14-item semantic-differential scale developed by Atchley (1974). Items assessing overall health rating, health trend, functional capacity, and activity limitation were adapted from questions used in the National Health Interview Survey. An adapted form of Lawton's (1975) Philadelphia Geriatric Center Morale Scale was used to assess morale (Morris and Sherwood 1975). The measure used to assess ADL/IADL status was adapted from survey instruments commonly used in long-term care assessment. Marital satisfaction was measured using a scale developed by Gilford and Bengtson (1979), which taps the frequency of both positive and negative experiences in a marriage.

Other scales were constructed and validated in pilot studies for use in this research, including scales of retirement beliefs, activity level, personal goal directedness, and self-confidence, which were used across all waves of the study. For 1995, two new scales were included: a gerotranscendence scale adapted from a scale developed by Tornstam (1994) and a continuity scale developed by Atchley. All of these scales displayed sufficient reliability in pretests, and subsequent tests of internal reliability have been quite satisfactory.

Fifteen drafts of the 1975 OLSAA questionnaire were field tested before the final 1975 version was established. In addition, information learned from early waves of the research was used to refine subsequent questionnaires. Although most of the key items remained the same throughout all six waves of data collection, some revisions were made to improve data quality. For example, Lawton's original morale scale used a simple yes/no format for 17 of the 21 scale items. Many of the 1975 respondents were unhappy with the categorical nature of this format. In subsequent waves, we used a four-choice Likert format (strongly agree, agree, disagree, strongly disagree) but scored the responses dichotomously, which produced scale scores generally comparable to those obtained using Lawton's format. The Likert format increased the reliability of the scale, reduced the amount of missing data within the scale, and reduced written comments qualifying responses to the scale. Being able to express their degree of agreement or disagreement was important to the respondents.

The questionnaire used in the 1995 wave of the study is reproduced in Appendix C.

Data Collection and Data Management

Data collection began in early October 1975 to allow most of the data to be collected before Thanksgiving. Questionnaires were mailed to 1,858 people whose names and addresses had been identified as comprising the target population. Because several methods of identification were used to identify panel members, different spellings of names or combinations of initials made it difficult in some cases to determine whether we had one respondent or two in the household. For example, was Mrs. Howard Johnson, S. J. Johnson, and Jane Johnson, all listed for the same address, the same person, two different people, or three different people? In many cases we could resolve these issues by using community informants, but in cases where we could not, the study team decided to err on the side of including more than one name when a seeming ambiguity could not be resolved. This means, of course, that we are unable to say with certainty that the names and addresses that comprised the initial mailing list contained no unduplicated persons. Likewise, we could not be sure exactly what the effective base number should be for calculating the survey response rate. As mentioned earlier, we were able to establish later an intercensal estimate of the target population of 1,805, which suggests that the original mailing list contained about 50 duplications.

Two weeks after the initial mailing, a reminder postcard was mailed to each prospect who had not yet returned a questionnaire; at one month, a second questionnaire was sent to those who had not yet responded, and at six weeks, another reminder postcard was sent. Those who still had not replied by eight weeks were contacted by telephone or in person. All but six people in the target population responded or were personally contacted. Twenty-three in-person interviews were conducted, mostly with respondents who were blind or had low vision. Persons with dementia were excluded from the study. These extensive efforts to secure participation resulted in completed questionnaires from 1,106 respondents, a response rate of about 61 percent. Of the responses received, 997 (55%) consisted of responses to nearly all items on the questionnaire.

The response rate would have been higher had it not been for the historical accident of when the study was conducted relative to the development of human-subject standards by the National Institutes of Health. Rocked by a series of scandals concerning abuse of human subjects in funded research, the NIH responded by subjecting all funded research to very intrusive human-subject protocols. The OLSAA was required to obtain signed consent forms from each respondent, even though the survey was completely voluntary and asked no questions about immoral or illegal behavior. We estimate that the requirement to get signatures reduced the response rate by at least 10 percent. By the time of the second wave, signatures were no longer required, and 165 potential respondents who had not responded to the first wave entered the study at that time, which increased the response rate to at least one of the first two surveys to 70.5 percent.

Data were coded, checked, and cleaned using standard survey data management procedures such as contingency cleaning and possible code cleaning (Babbie 1995), and computer programs were written to generate scale scores. The data were then organized into a computer file formatted for analysis using the SPSS data management and statistical analysis computer software package. SPSS was chosen because at that time it had contingency table column and row labeling capabilities superior to those available in comparable software.

The population was resurveyed using these same procedures in 1977, 1979, and 1981, at which time NIMH funding of the data collection effort ended. Returns were 852, 678, and 667, respectively. Effective response rates to the follow-up waves ranged from 75 to 80 percent. More than 200 of the original respondents had died by 1981. An unknown number of refusals resulted from increases in the prevalence of cognitive impairment as the study population aged.

The study population contained a large number of married couples with both members in the study population, and both members of 210 couples completed questionnaires for the 1975 and 1977 waves. A separate couples file was created to allow easier analysis of data using the couple as the unit of analysis. There were 68 intact couples remaining in the study in 1995. This represents one of the best existing longitudinal records of data from both members of couples in middle and later life.

In 1991, with funding from the Ohio Long-Term Care Research Project, the OLSAA panel was again resurveyed employing the same procedures used to collect earlier waves. Questionnaires were sent to all people who had responded to at least two earlier waves. Because of the 10-year interval since the last wave of data had been collected, extensive efforts were needed to identify those who had died and to track down respondents who had moved. Only two respondents could not be found. The 1991 questionnaire was sent to a total of 623 people, and we received back 474, a response rate of 76 percent. In 1995, questionnaires were sent to 423 respondents from at least three waves of the study, including 1991, with completed returns of 309, a response rate of 73 percent.

The data for all waves were organized into an integrated six-wave longitudinal file that included all those who responded to any of the OLSAA surveys. This file is archived at Miami University and at the Henry Murray Research Center at Radcliffe College.

The 1995 Study Questionnaire

1. Is the person to whom this questionnaire is addressed physically and mentally able to complete the questionnaire?

   ☐ Yes. Please go to Question 2.

   ☐ No. Please return this questionnaire in the enclosed envelope. Thank you.

2. How many years have you lived at your current address? _____

3. What is your sex?

   ☐ Male

   ☐ Female

4. What is your date of birth?

   Month _____ Year _____

5. Are you retired?

   ☐ Yes. At what age did you retire?_____
   Please skip to Question 7.

   ☐ No

6. Do you plan to retire?

   ☐ Yes. At what age do you plan to retire? _____

   ☐ No

   ☐ Don't know

   ☐ Does not apply; have not had a paid job to retire from.

1

7. Is your spouse retired? (If you are not presently married, skip to Question 9.)

☐ Yes. At what age did your spouse retire?_____
   Please skip to Question 9.

☐ No

8. Does your spouse plan to retire?

☐ Yes. At what age does he or she plan to retire? _____

☐ No

☐ Don't know

☐ Does not apply; has not had a paid job that he or she can retire from.

9. The purpose of the following items is to see how people rate their lives in retirement on a series of opposites. Make your judgements on the basis of what you think YOUR LIFE IN RETIREMENT **is** or **will be** like.

The **EXAMPLE** below shows how to use the sets of opposites.

If you feel that
YOUR LIFE IN
RETIREMENT
is or will be: You should mark:

	extremely	quite	slightly	neutral	slightly	quite	extremely	
QUITE SICK	sick		✔					healthy
NEITHER GOOD NOR BAD	good				✔			bad
EXTREMELY ACTIVE	active	✔						inactive

Now, go to the top of the next page and begin to mark sets of opposites.

2

IMPORTANT (1) Be sure you check how you would rate each and every pair of opposites – **do not omit any.**

(2) Never put more than one mark for a single set of opposites.

YOUR LIFE IN RETIREMENT

Below is a list of adjectives that can be used to describe a person's life. For each line, check the ONE box that best describes what you think about **your life in retirement** – about how your life **is** or **will be** during your retirement.

	extremely	quite	slightly	neutral	slightly	quite	extremely	
sick								healthy
good								bad
active								inactive
sad								happy
immobile								mobile
involved								uninvolved
unable								able
dependent								independent
hopeful								hopeless
worthy								worthless
satisfied								dissatisfied
full								empty
busy								idle
meaningful								meaningless

START HERE ☞

3

10. Next is a series of statements about retirement. In the spaces provided, please indicate the extent to which you think these statements apply to **retired people in general.**

Mark only **one** answer for **each** statement.

	almost none	a few	many	almost all
Retirement causes people to get sick.				
Retirement leads to premature death.				
When people retire, they miss their jobs.				
When people retire, they lose touch with who they are.				
Retirement causes people to age more rapidly.				
Retirement is a difficult adjustment.				
Retirement causes people to suffer mental problems.				
Retired people have trouble finding things to do.				
When people retire, they lose contact with their friends.				

11. What is your **primary** means of transportation?

☐ Driver, private auto   ☐ Walking

☐ Passenger, private auto   ☐ HELP Van

☐ Taxicab   ☐ Other (Please specify)

_____

_____

4

These next few questions concern your health and general physical well-being.

12. How would you rate your health? (Mark only one answer.)

☐ Very Good ☐ Good ☐ Fair ☐ Poor ☐ Very Poor

13. In this section, we are interested in how frequently you have performed these activities in the last **twenty years**. Review each item below and check **how often** you performed that type of activity. (Mark only one answer per item.)

Had a complete physical examination at least every three years.

☐ Always ☐ Usually ☐ Sometimes ☐ Seldom ☐ Never

Ate a balance diet with a restricted fat intake.

☐ Always ☐ Usually ☐ Sometimes ☐ Seldom ☐ Never

Attempted to maintain a desired weight, avoiding overweight or underweight.

☐ Always ☐ Usually ☐ Sometimes ☐ Seldom ☐ Never

Used a car seatbelt.

☐ Always ☐ Usually ☐ Sometimes ☐ Seldom ☐ Never

Participated in some type of exercise.

☐ Always ☐ Usually ☐ Sometimes ☐ Seldom ☐ Never

Limited your alcohol consumption.

☐ Always ☐ Usually ☐ Sometimes ☐ Seldom ☐ Never

Avoided or eliminated use of tobacco. (i.e., cigarettes, pipes, chewing tobacco).

☐ Always ☐ Usually ☐ Sometimes ☐ Seldom ☐ Never

Followed the directions for taking prescription medications.

☐ Always ☐ Usually ☐ Sometimes ☐ Seldom ☐ Never

5

14. How often do you have trouble sleeping? (Mark only one answer.)

☐ Almost never

☐ Seldom

☐ Sometimes

☐ Often

☐ Nearly always

15. In general, would you say that over the past year or so your health has improved, declined, or remained about the same?

☐ Improved

☐ Declined

☐ Remained about the same

16. Which of the following things are you PHYSICALLY able to do?
(Place a check by **EACH** of the things you can do.)

☐ Heavy work around the house (shoveling snow, washing walls, etc.).

☐ Work at a full-time job.

☐ Do ordinary work around the house.

☐ Walk half a mile.

☐ Go out to a movie, to church, to a meeting or to visit.

☐ Walk up and down stairs.

17. Are your activities limited by health or disability?

☐ No limitation. (If you marked no limitation, skip to Question 20.)

☐ Some limitation, but not major activities such as employment or ordinary work around the house.

☐ Some limitation in amount or kind of major activities.

☐ Unable to carry on major activities.

18. Which of your activities are limited?

_____

_____

_____

_____

_____

19. What is the cause of your limitation?

_____

_____

_____

_____

_____

7

20. In this section we are interested in how you spend your time, the kinds of things you do when you are not on the job. Below, we have provided a list of the types of things many people do. We would like you to examine each item on this list, and indicate **how often** you engage in that kind of activity. (Mark only one answer per item.)

_____ Watching television or listening to radio.

□ very often □ often □ sometimes □ seldom □ very seldom □ never

_____ Gardening and /or care of animals and plants.

□ very often □ often □ sometimes □ seldom □ very seldom □ never

_____ Outdoor activities: camping, hiking, fishing, hunting, boating, etc.

□ very often □ often □ sometimes □ seldom □ very seldom □ never

_____ Participatory art: such as, playing a musical instrument, painting pictures, being in plays, photography, etc.

□ very often □ often □ sometimes □ seldom □ very seldom □ never

_____ Spectator art: going to plays, operas, ballet, museums, musical performances, etc.

□ very often □ often □ sometimes □ seldom □ very seldom □ never

_____ Exercising: fitness walking, aerobics, swimming, weight training, etc.

□ very often □ often □ sometimes □ seldom □ very seldom □ never

_____ Handiwork: metal work, woodworking, embroidery, sewing, knitting, pottery making, etc.

□ very often □ often □ sometimes □ seldom □ very seldom □ never

_____ Participatory sports: playing tennis, golfing, bowling, etc.

□ very often □ often □ sometimes □ seldom □ very seldom □ never

_____ Household work: laundry, lawn mowing, washing dishes, home repairs, etc.

□ very often □ often □ sometimes □ seldom □ very seldom □ never

_____ Collecting: stamp collecting, coin collecting, rock collecting, antique collecting, etc.

☐ very often ☐ often ☐ sometimes ☐ seldom ☐ very seldom ☐ never

_____ Participating in games such as bridge, chess, checkers, dominoes, etc.

☐ very often ☐ often ☐ sometimes ☐ seldom ☐ very seldom ☐ never

_____ Participating in elections and political activities (other than voting).

☐ very often ☐ often ☐ sometimes ☐ seldom ☐ very seldom ☐ never

_____ Cooking or baking.

☐ very often ☐ often ☐ sometimes ☐ seldom ☐ very seldom ☐ never

_____ Reading.

☐ very often ☐ often ☐ sometimes ☐ seldom ☐ very seldom ☐ never

_____ Participating in the activities of farm organizations, labor unions, or professional groups.

☐ very often ☐ often ☐ sometimes ☐ seldom ☐ very seldom ☐ never

_____ Outings: non-food shopping, eating at restaurants, going to movies, etc.

☐ very often ☐ often ☐ sometimes ☐ seldom ☐ very seldom ☐ never

_____ Participating in the activities of lodges, social clubs, civic associations, or community service organizations.

☐ very often ☐ often ☐ sometimes ☐ seldom ☐ very seldom ☐ never

_____ Participating in the activities of senior citizens' organizations.

☐ very often ☐ often ☐ sometimes ☐ seldom ☐ very seldom ☐ never

_____ Resting: taking a nap, contemplating, relaxing, etc.

☐ very often ☐ often ☐ sometimes ☐ seldom ☐ very seldom ☐ never

9

_____ Spectator sports: going to see **(not watching on television)** football, baseball, wrestling, racing, etc.

☐	☐	☐	☐	☐	☐
very often	often	sometimes	seldom	very seldom	never

_____ Traveling.

☐	☐	☐	☐	☐	☐
very often	often	sometimes	seldom	very seldom	never

_____ Being with neighbors or friends.

☐	☐	☐	☐	☐	☐
very often	often	sometimes	seldom	very seldom	never

_____ Being with children and grandchildren.

☐	☐	☐	☐	☐	☐
very often	often	sometimes	seldom	very seldom	never

_____ Being with relatives other than children and grandchildren.

☐	☐	☐	☐	☐	☐
very often	often	sometimes	seldom	very seldom	never

_____ Organized social gatherings: parties or get-togethers.

☐	☐	☐	☐	☐	☐
very often	often	sometimes	seldom	very seldom	never

_____ Helping family members or friends: baby-sitting, home repairs, shopping, providing transportation, cooking, etc.

☐	☐	☐	☐	☐	☐
very often	often	sometimes	seldom	very seldom	never

_____ Participating in volunteer activities.

☐	☐	☐	☐	☐	☐
very often	often	sometimes	seldom	very seldom	never

_____ Attending church functions.

☐	☐	☐	☐	☐	☐
very often	often	sometimes	seldom	very seldom	never

STOP. Now go back to the beginning of the above list on page 8, and place a check on the line to the left of **each** kind of activity that you would like to do more often.

10

21. In the spaces below please list the **five** activities you do most often.
(You do not have to use the same categories as those given in the preceding list.)

1. _____

2. _____

3. _____

4. _____

5. _____

22. Overall, how satisfied would you say you are with the way you spend your time?

☐ Very Satisfied   ☐ Satisfied   ☐ Unsatisfied   ☐ Very Unsatisfied

23. Are you satisfied with the amount of free time you have now, or do you feel you have too much free time or too little free time?

☐ Too little free time

☐ Satisfied with the amount of free time

☐ Too much free time

11

24. Next we are interested in finding out the kinds of things that are important to people, the kinds of things that give their lives meaning – their personal goals. Below, we have provided a list of very general kinds of things that some people define as their personal goals. We would like you to read through that list, and rate how important or unimportant each goal is in your life. (Mark only one answer per goal.)

	Very Important	Important	Unimportant	Very Unimportant
_____ Being well-read and informed.				
_____ Having close ties with my family.				
_____ Being prominent in community affairs.				
_____ Having a substantial income.				
_____ Having a satisfying job.				
_____ Forming close, long-lasting friendships.				
_____ Being self-reliant and self-sufficient.				
_____ Seeking new experiences and opportunities.				
_____ Having a comfortable place to live.				
_____ Having roots in the community.				
_____ Being seen as a good person by others.				
_____ Being dependable and reliable.				
_____ Being accepted by influential people.				
_____ Being a religious person.				
_____ Having a close, intimate relationship with another person.				
_____ Being able to accept myself as I am.				
_____ Doing things for others				

STOP. Now look back to the beginning of the list, and indicate, in the spaces provided to the left of the goals, which ones you associate with your job or working. (If you are a housewife, mark the goals which you associate with your housework; if your are retired, mark the goals which you used to associate with your job or working before you retired.)

25. Please list your five most important goals IN ORDER OF THEIR IMPORTANCE. Feel free to use your own words and do not feel limited by the goals listed on the preceding page.

1. _____ (MOST IMPORTANT)

2. _____

3. _____

4. _____

5. _____ (LEAST IMPORTANT)

26. The next set of questions asks you to compare yourself today with yourself when you were age 50. (Mark only one answer per item.)

Compared to when I was 50:

	Strongly Agree	Agree	Disagree	Strongly Disagree
Death seems less frightening.				
I feel a greater connection with the entire universe.				
I take myself more seriously.				
Material things generally mean more to me.				
I take more enjoyment from my inner life.				
I feel less connection with both past and future generations.				

What enables you to cope? What keeps you going?

_____

_____

_____

_____

_____

13

There are a few things we would like to know about your employment experiences.

27. First, what is your present employment status?
(Check the **one** category that **best** describes your situation.)

☐ Housewife, no paid employment

☐ Housewife, retired from paid employment

☐ Retired, not working

☐ Retired, working part-time

☐ Retired, working full-time

☐ Employed, part-time

☐ Employed, full-time

☐ Unemployed

28. What is or was your specific job title? (Use the title of your last job if you are unemployed or retired.) _____

Briefly describe your duties. _____

_____

_____

(If you are not employed, skip to Question 30.)

29. How many hours per week do you work? _____

How many weeks per year do you work? _____

14

30. How do you feel about your work?
    (If your are **retired**, how did you feel about your work?)
    (Mark only one answer.)

    ☐ Strongly enjoy it

    ☐ Generally enjoy it

    ☐ Sometimes enjoy it, sometimes not

    ☐ Generally dislike it

    ☐ Strongly dislike it

31. Have you (or did you) consciously set goals that you wanted to achieve through your work: things like being the best machinist in the shop, or being the best scholar in your field, or simply being good at your job?

    ☐ No

    ☐ Yes   If "yes", to what extent do you feel that you have met those goals?
            (Mark only one answer.)

           ☐ Met

           ☐ Partially met

           ☐ Unmet

32. As I get older, things are (better, worse, or the same) as I thought they would be.

    ☐ Better   ☐ Worse   ☐ The same

33. If you could live where you wanted, where would you live?

    ☐ In this community   ☐ Some place else

15

34. How much do you feel lonely?

    ☐ Not much   ☐ A lot

35. How satisfied are you with your life today?

    ☐ Satisfied   ☐ Not satisfied

Sometimes people are not able to perform certain activities without assistance because of ill health or disability. We are interested in whether you have provided or received such assistance on a regular basis because of **ill health or disability.** Some examples of activities requiring assistance include help with regular household chores, cooking, shopping, transportation, or personal care (such as bathing or dressing).

36. Do you now **provide** or have you in the past 10 years **provided** assistance for an extended period of time to someone inside or outside your household because of their ill health or disability? (Check all that apply.)

    ☐ Yes, I provide(d) such assistance to someone **inside** my household.

    ☐ Yes, I provide(d) such assistance to someone **outside** my household.

    ☐ No, I have not provided such assistance during the past 10 years.

37. Do you now **receive** or have you in the past 10 years **received** assistance for an extended period of time from someone inside or outside your household because of your ill health or disability? (Check all that apply.)

    ☐ Yes, I receive(d) such assistance from someone **inside** my household.

    ☐ Yes, I receive(d) such assistance from someone **outside** my household.

    ☐ No, I have not received such assistance during the past 10 years.

16

38. Next is a series of items designed to see how life has been for you recently. In the spaces provided, indicate how much you agree or disagree with each item.

(Mark only one answer per item.)

	Strongly Agree	Agree	Disagree	Strongly Disagree
I am as happy now as I was when I was younger.				
I have as much pep as I did last year.				
I sometimes worry so much that I can't sleep.				
Little things bother me more this year.				
I see enough of my friends and relatives.				
As you get older, you are less useful.				
I sometimes feel that life isn't worth living.				
Things keep getting worse as I get older.				
Most days I have plenty to do.				
Life is hard for me most of the time.				
I have a lot to be sad about.				
People had it better in the old days.				
I am afraid of a lot of things.				
I get mad more than I used to.				
I take things hard.				
A person has to live for today and not worry about tomorrow.				
I get upset easily.				

17

39. Following is a list of home management, personal care, and daily activities. Please tell us whether you are **PHYSICALLY AND MENTALLY** able to do each of these activities, independently or with some kind of assistance. We are not asking whether you actually do these activities, but whether you would physically and mentally be able to do them.

(Mark only one answer for each item.)	Can do without help from another person	Can do only with help of another person	Unable to do this activity
Do heavy work around the house (shovel snow, washing walls, etc.)			
Do light housework (dusting, vacuuming, etc.)			
Prepare meals			
Go shopping			
Manage money			
Use the telephone			
Take a bath or shower			
Get dressed			
Eat			
Get in and out of a chair or bed			
Get outside			
Use the toilet			
Walk around the block			
Walk around inside the house			

18

40. For these questions, we are interested in your general impressions or opinions. Make a check to show how much you agree or disagree with each of the following statements as they apply to you now. (Mark only one answer per statement.)

	Strongly Agree	Agree	Disagree	Strongly Disagree
I can do just about anything that I set my mind to.				
I am a go-getter.				
My life seems doomed to failure.				
I am afraid to talk to people in authority.				
If I want something, I go out and get it.				
I have trouble talking to people about myself.				
Often I do not really make decisions; I just let things happen.				
When I need to solve problems, I usually try solutions that have worked for me before.				
I know myself well enough to know which choices are best for me.				
Over the years, I have continued activities that suit me and discontinued ones that do not.				
My choices seldom turn out as well as I expect.				
I have no sense of the direction I want my life to take.				
My philosophy of life is a consistent force behind the decisions I make.				
My basic lifestyle has changed significantly in the past 10 years.				
Most of my friends are people I first met within the past 10 years.				
My basic beliefs and values have change significantly in the past 10 years.				

(If you are not now married skip to Question 44.)

19

41. Please read the following list of some things husbands and wives may do when they are together. Please indicate how often it happens between you and your spouse.

(Mark only one answer for each item.)	Hardly ever	Not usually, but sometimes	Fairly Often	Quite frequently	Always
You calmly discuss something					
One of you is sarcastic					
You work together on something (dishes, yardwork, hobbies, etc.)					
One of you refuses to talk in a normal manner					
You laugh together					
You have a stimulating exchange of ideas					
You disagree about something important					
You become critical or belittling					
You have a good time together					
You become angry					

42. All things considered, how satisfied are you with your marriage overall?

☐ Extremely satisfied ☐ Satisfied ☐ Dissatisfied ☐ Extremely dissatisfied

20

43. What changes do you anticipate retirement will make or what changes did it make in the quality of your relationship with your spouse?

_____

_____

_____

_____

_____

44. Not counting yourself, how many people LIVE IN YOUR HOUSEHOLD more than six months a year? _____

The following question refers only to those people who LIVE IN YOUR HOUSEHOLD. How are the people who LIVE IN YOUR HOUSEHOLD related to you (spouse, child, brother, friend, etc.)?

	Age	Relationship to you
Person #1	_____	_____
Person #2	_____	_____
Person #3	_____	_____
Person #4	_____	_____
Person #5	_____	_____
Person #6	_____	_____

45. **Not counting the people in your own household**, how many of your close **friends** live within thirty-five miles of you? (Mark only one answer.)

☐ none ☐ 1-5 ☐ 6-15 ☐ 16-25 ☐ more than 25

46. **Not counting the people in your own household**, how many of your close **relatives** live within thirty-five miles of you? (Mark only one answer.)

☐ none ☐ 1-5 ☐ 6-15 ☐ 16-25 ☐ more than 25

21

This final set of questions is designed to provide us with a general picture of the people in our study.

47. Do you consider your present family or household income enough to meet your living expenses?

☐ Yes

☐ No

48. How much monthly income would you say your household needs just to get by?

_____

49. Into which of the following categories does your year pre-tax household income fall?

☐ less than $5,000   ☐ $30,000 to $39,999

☐ $5,000 to $9,999   ☐ $40,000 to $49,999

☐ $10,000 to $19,999   ☐ $50,000 to $59,999

☐ $20,000 to $29,999   ☐ $60,000 to $69,999

                                      ☐ More than $70,000

50. Do you have living children?

☐ No

☐ Yes

If "yes"   how many sons? _____ what ages? _____

                 how many daughters? _____ what ages? _____

51. What is your **current** marital status? **(Mark only one answer.)**

    ☐ Never married

    ☐ Widowed   (How many years have you been widowed? _____)

    ☐ Separated   (How many years have you been separated?_____)

    ☐ Divorced   (How many years have you been divorced? _____)

    ☐ Married   (How old is your spouse? _____)

                       (How many years have you been married

                       to your current spouse? _____)

52. Is the address on the front of the envelope your current address?

    ☐ Yes

    ☐ If no, what is your current address?

    _____

    _____

    _____

53. Would you please give us the name and address of a close family member or friend who is likely to always know where to contact you?

    _____

    _____

    _____

Surveys such as ours often seem impersonal. Because we have a large number of people participating, we have to anticipate your answers to some extent. Otherwise we would never be able to put the results together into an overall picture. But what is missing from these very structured items is the personal touch, the meaningful details that put your answers in context.

For all of those topics about which you thought "yes, but" or "I agree, except" or "let me explain...", and for those questions you thought we should have asked and didn't, please feel free to write comments in the space on these pages. We have learned a lot from your comments over the years, and we encourage you to express yourself if you feel like it.

THANK YOU ONCE AGAIN FOR PARTICIPATING IN OUR STUDY.

NOW TAKE THE QUESTIONNAIRE, FOLD IT IN HALF (TOP TO BOTTOM), AND PUT

IT INSIDE THE SELF-ADDRESSED, POSTPAID ENVELOPE WHICH WAS INCLUDED

WITH THE MATERIALS YOU RECEIVED. THEN SEAL THE ENVELOPE AND MAIL IT.

THE POSTAGE HAS ALREADY BEEN PAID. DO NOT AFFIX A STAMP.

24

Worksheets Used to Examine
Longitudinal Patterns

In analyzing the data for several waves of data collection, especially with unequal intervals between waves, traditional statistical procedures are unable to handle what amounts to a multivariate time series analysis. If we want to look at patterns of continuity and discontinuity in the context of other patterns, statistical modeling tools such as LISREL or EQS are fine for two waves of data, but they cannot be used with several waves. But perhaps more importantly, looking at time trends both in summary measures and in detailed items simultaneously works better if the investigator has some sort of visual display that allows patterns to be classified and compared.

Worksheet 1 is an example of how an enormous amount of longitudinal data can be displayed for each case record. In row 1, at the top of the page, the respondent's identification number, gender, age in 1995, education, and race are displayed, along with summary scale scores for behavioral rigidity, disposition toward continuity, gerotranscendence, and preventive health practices.

The first block of longitudinal results shows marital status, marital satisfaction scale score, self-confidence scale score, activity level, functional capability score, self-rated health, perceived health trend, goal directedness scale score, morale scale score, life in retirement rating scale score, social withdrawal scale score, score on adequacy of sleep, and beliefs about retirement. The vertical line indicates the beginning of the individual items contained in the morale scale. The remaining morale items continue into block 2 and end at the vertical line. The remainder of block 2 consists of individual items that make up the self-confidence scale.

Block 3 consists of the individual items in the life in retirement rating scale. Block 4 consists of individual items in the activity inventory, which continues into block 5 for the first five columns. Then block 5 lists individual items for the functional capability scale, activity limitation scale score, and ADL/IADL items, which continue into block 6 for the first nine columns.

The remainder of block 6 consists of scores on receiving assistance, principal modes of transportation, and the first ten individual items of the personal goals scale.

Block 7 continues the personal goals items for the first seven columns followed by scores on the Gilford and Bengtson marital satisfaction scale and scores on the individual items (these items were present for only 1991 and 1995).

Block 8 contains the number of persons in the respondent's household, respondent's number of living children, number of relatives living in the community, and number of friends living in the community. Block 8 continues with occupation, employment/retirement status, scale score on attitude toward work, income adequacy, years at current address, income, number of pensions currently being drawn, number of eventual pensions, number of public employer pensions, number of private pensions, and social security or railroad retirement pensions.

In all, Worksheet 1 potentially displays 842 pieces of information in a format that allows visual inspection of the degree of continuity and discontinuity over time.

Worksheet 2 displays coded answers to open-ended questions such as occupation, hours and weeks worked per year, amount and cause of disability, type of assistance received, and amount of income needed just to get by. It also contains the respondents' own statements of personal goals and activities, whether they help others, and if so, whom. Finally, Worksheet 2 displays the age and relationship to another person in the household and the coded answers to the open-ended questions concerning how respondents cope.

In combination, Worksheets 1 and 2 provide a wealth of information in very compact form. Color coding was used to identify different shapes of trends and patterns. I used these worksheets extensively in selecting specific respondents for in-depth interviews and for constructing case histories. Worksheets 1 and 2 were done for all respondents to wave 6 of data collection.

Worksheet 3 is an example of those used to tabulate patterns of response to specific questionnaire items, in this case frequency of participation in a specific activity category. As the worksheet shows, there were a great many possible patterns, and nearly all of the possible patterns were observed. This type of analysis gets at the variations *within* patterns such as stability, continuity, and discontinuity.

These worksheets aid what I call the qualitative analysis of mostly quantitative data. This type of analysis is crucial for an understanding of how patterns of ideas or life dimensions relate to one another in a holistic framework. Such analyses allow the investigator to get a sense of how the personal construct space of each individual is organized and how it changed over time, for in the end, when researchers ask questions, the answers received are framed by the personal constructs of the respondents, even for seemingly close-ended questions.

WORKSHEET 1

ID: Sex: Age6:   Ed: Race: Ret.Age: Rigid: Cont: G-T: PrHlt:

	Mst	Msat	S-C	Act.	Fhlt	Hlt	Htrd	Gols	PGC	SmD	wthd	slep	strty		wrse	pep	both	fam	less	wliv	hapy
1975																					
1977																					
1979																					
1981																					
1991																					
1995																					

	plnty	sad	betr	fraid	mad	tkhd	tday	same	live	lnly	satf	wrry	lifh	upst		anyt	gogt	doom	frai	getit	talk	
1975																						
1977																						
1979																						
1981																						
1991																						
1995																						

	sick	bad	inac	sad	imob	uninv	unab	indp	hpls	wthls	dsat	emty	idle	meang	
1975															
1977															
1979															
1981															
1991															
1995															

	gard	part	sart	hand	pspt	coll	pgam	polor	ocor	comor	ssprt	trav	frnd	chld	read	TV	gath	chrch	senor	rest
1975																				
1977																				
1979																				
1981																				
1991																				
1995																				

	help	outg	frsat	frtim	prast		hvyw	flxmw	orwk	walk	goout	stair	aclim	ADL	hvyw	ltwk	meal	shop	$
1975																			
1977																			
1979																			
1981																			
1991																			
1995																			

	phon	bath	dres	eat	trsf	otsd	tlet	bloc	insd		reast	trnsp		info	famr	prom	incm	job	frnd	srel	nexp	comf	root
1975																							
1977																							
1979																							
1981																							
1991																							
1995																							

	gdpn	rebl	accp	rel	inti	acsel	dofr		mscal	disc	sarc	wktg	mute	lagh	exch	dsag	crit	gtim	angr	
1975																				
1977																				
1979																				
1981																				
1991																				
1995																				

	nhous	nmkd	rels	fnds	occ	empl	wkatd	adinc	yrcad	incm	curpen	evpen	prp	evprp	ssrr
1975															
1977															
1979															
1981															
1991															
1995															

WORKSHEET 2

ID: Sex: Age6:   Educ:

1977	Job2:					
1979	Job3:		hrswk:	wksyr:		
1981	Job4		hrswk:	wksyr:		
1991	Job5		hrswk:	wksyr:		

1981	Disblty	Whylim				
1991	Disblty5	Whylim5			Recasst5	Getby5
1995	Disblty6	Why6lim1	Why6lim2	Why6lim3	Recasst6	Getby6

1979					Retchng	Yeschng
1981	Rankgol1	Rankgol2	Rankgol3	Rankgol4	T4changs	
1991	Rank1g5	Rank2g5	Rank3g5	Rank4g5	T5changs	othrchg5
1995	Rank1g6	Rank2g6	Rank3g6	Rank4g6	T6changs	othrghg6

1981	Freqact1	Frreqact2	Freqact3	Freqact4	Freqact5	yrmarrd4
1991	Frq5act1	Frq5act2	Frq5act3	Frq5act4	Frq5act5	yrmarrd5
1995	Frq6act1	Frq6act2	Frq6act3	Frq6act4	Frq6act5	yrmarrd6

| 1991 | Proasst5 | othrhelp | finrspn | age5per1 | t5persn1 | |
| 1995 | Proasst6 | whohelp | whofinsu | age6per1 | t5persn1 | |

Howcope1   Howcope2   Howcope3   Howcope4   Howcope5

WORKSHEET 3

Variable:

Stable   6_____
5_____
4_____
3_____
2_____
1_____

Continuity 6-_____6/5_____
5/6_____5+_____5-_____
5/4_____4/5_____
4+_____4-_____4/3_____3/4_____
3+_____3-_____
3/2_____
1/2_____

Discontinuity
U   _ 4 _ _____
_ 3 _ _____
_ 2 _ _____
_ 1 _ _____

Inv. U   _6_ _____
_5_ _____
_4_ _____

\   6-4_____6-3_____6-2_____6-1_____
5-3_____5-2_____5-1_____
4-2_____4-1_____
3-1_____

/   4-6_____3-6_____2-6_____1-6_____
3-5_____2-5_____1-5_____
2-4_____1-4_____
1-3_____

W   _____

M   _____

Other _____

| References

Achenbaum, Andrew W., and Lucinda Orwoll. 1991. Becoming wise: Psychological interpretation of the Book of Job. *International Journal of Aging and Human Development* 32:21–39.

Alexander, Charles N., John L. Davies, Carol A. Dixon, Michael C. Dillbeck, Steven M. Drucker, Roberta M. Oetzel, John M. Muehlman, and David W. Orme-Johnson. 1990. Growth of higher stages of consciousness: Maharishi's Vedic psychology of human development. In C. N. Alexander and E. J. Langer (eds.), *Higher Stages of Adult Development.* New York: Oxford University Press, pp. 286–341.

Antonucci, Toni C. 1990. Social supports and social relationships. In R. H. Binstock and L. K. George (eds.), *Handbook of Aging and the Social Sciences,* 3d ed. New York: Academic Press, pp. 205–26.

Atchley, Robert C. 1967. "Retired Women: A Study of Self and Role." Ph.D. diss., Washington, D.C.: The American University.

———. 1969. Respondents vs. refusers in an interview study of retired women. *Journal of Gerontology* 24:42–47.

———. 1971a. Retirement and leisure participation: Continuity or crisis? *Gerontologist* 11:13–17.

———. 1971b. Disengagement among professors. *Journal of Gerontology* 26:476–80.

———. 1971c. Retirement and work orientation. *Gerontologist* 11:29–32.

———. 1974. The meaning of retirement. *Journal of Communications* 24(4):97–101.

———. 1975a. The life course, age grading, and age-linked demands for decision making. In N. Datan and L. H. Ginsberg (eds.), *Life-Span Developmental Psychology: Normative Life Crises.* New York: Academic Press, pp. 261–78.

———. 1975b. Adjustment to loss of job at retirement. *International Journal of Aging and Human Development* 6:17–27.

———. 1976a. Orientation toward the job and retirement adjustment among women. In J. F. Gubrium (ed.), *Time, Self, and Aging.* New York: Behavioral Publications, pp. 199–208.

———. 1976b. Selected social and psychological differences between men and women in later life. *Journal of Gerontology* 31:204–11.

———. 1976c. *Sociology of Retirement.* Cambridge, Mass.: Schenkman.

——. 1979. Issues in retirement research. *Gerontologist* 19:44–54.

——. 1982a. Retirement: Leaving the world of work. *Annals of the American Academy of Political and Social Sciences* 464:120–31.

——. 1982b. The process of retirement: Comparing women and men. In M. Szinovacz (ed.), *Women's Retirement.* Beverly Hills, Calif.: Sage, pp. 153–68.

——. 1982c. The aging self. *Psychotherapy: Theory, Research, and Practice* 19:388–96.

——. 1985. *Social Forces and Aging,* 4th ed. Belmont, Calif.: Wadsworth.

——. 1989. A continuity theory of normal aging. *Gerontologist* 29:183–90.

——. 1991. The influence of aging and frailty on perceptions and expressions of the self. In J. E. Birren et al. (eds.), *The Concept and Measurement of Quality of Life in the Frail Elderly.* New York: Academic Press, pp. 207–25.

——. 1993. Continuity theory and the evolution of activity in later life. In J. R. Kelly (ed.), *Activity and Aging.* Newbury Park, Calif.: Sage, pp. 5–16

——. 1995. Continuity theory. In G. L. Maddox et al. (eds.), *Encyclopedia of Aging,* 2d ed. New York: Springer, pp. 227–30.

——. 1996. Continuity of the spiritual self. In M. Kimble et al. (eds.), *Religion, Spirituality and Aging: A Handbook.* Minneapolis: Augsburg Fortress Press, pp. 68–73.

——. 1997a. Everyday mysticism: Spiritual development in later life. *Journal of Adult Development* 4:123–34.

——. 1997b. *Social Forces and Aging,* 8th ed. Belmont, Calif.: Wadsworth.

——. 1998. Activity adaptations to the development of functional limitations and results for subjective well-being: A qualitative analysis of longitudinal panel data over a 16-year period. *Journal of Aging Studies* 12:19–38.

Atchley, Robert C., and Linda K. George. 1973. Symptomatic measurement of age. *Gerontologist* 13:332–36.

Babbie, Earl R. 1995. *The Practice of Social Research,* 7th ed. Belmont, Calif.: Wadsworth.

Bailey, Kenneth D. 1990. *Social Entropy Theory.* Albany: State University of New York Press.

Baltes, Paul B. 1993. The aging mind: Potentials and limits. *Gerontologist* 33:580–94.

Becker, Gay. 1993. Continuity after a stroke: Implications of life-course disruption in old age. *Gerontologist* 33:148–58.

Bengtson, Vern L., Margaret N. Reedy, and Chad Gordon. 1985. Aging and self-conceptions: Personality processes and social contexts. In J. E. Birren and K. W. Schaie (eds.), *Handbook of the Psychology of Aging,* 2d ed. New York: Academic Press, pp. 544–93.

Bennett, Ruth G. 1980. *Aging, Isolation, and Resocialization.* New York: Van Nostrand Reinhold.

Biegel, David E., and Arthur Blum (eds.). 1990. *Aging and Caregiving: Theory, Research, and Policy.* Newbury Park, Calif.: Sage.

Bossé, Raymond, and Avron Spiro. 1995. Normative Aging Study. In G. L. Maddox et al. (eds.), *Encyclopedia of Aging,* 2d ed. New York: Springer, pp. 688–90.

Buckley, Walter. 1967. *Sociology and Modern Systems Theory*. Englewood Cliffs, N.J.: Prentice-Hall.

Carp, Frances M. 1968. Differences among older workers, volunteers, and persons who are neither. *Journal of Gerontology* 23:497–501.

Chow, Gilbert C. 1960. Tests of equality between sets of coefficients in two linear regressions. *Econometrica* 28:591–606.

Clark, Margaret, and Barbara Anderson. 1967. *Culture and Aging*. Springfield, Ill.: Charles C Thomas.

Cohler, Bertram. 1993. Aging, morale, and meaning: The nexus of narrative. In T. R. Cole, W. A. Achenbaum, P. L. Jakobi, and R. Kastenbaum (eds.), *Voices and Visions of Aging: Toward a Critical Gerontology*. New York: Springer, pp. 107–33.

Cumming, Elaine, and William E. Henry. 1961. *Growing Old: The Process of Disengagement*. New York: Basic Books.

Ekerdt, David. 1995. Retirement. In G. L. Maddox et al. (eds.), *Encyclopedia of Aging*, 2d ed. New York: Springer, pp. 819–23.

Epstein, Mark. 1995. *Thoughts Without a Thinker*. New York: Basic Books.

Erikson, Erik H. 1963. *Childhood and Society*. New York: Macmillan.

Erikson, Erik H., Joan M. Erikson, and Helen Q. Kivnick. 1986. *Vital Involvement in Old Age*. New York: Norton.

Fillenbaum, Gerda G. 1971. On the relation between attitude toward work and attitude toward retirement. *Journal of Gerontology* 24:244–48.

Fiske, Marjorie, and David A. Chiriboga. 1990. *Change and Continuity in Adult Life*. San Francisco: Jossey-Bass.

Friedmann, Eugene, and Robert J. Havighurst. 1954. *The Meaning of Work and Retirement*. Chicago: University of Chicago Press.

Gilford, Rosalie, and Vern L. Bengtson. 1979. Measuring marital satisfaction in three generations: Positive and negative dimensions. *Journal of Marriage and the Family* 41:387–98.

Greenwald, Anthony. 1980. The totalitarian ego: Fabrication and revision of personal history. *American Psychologist* 35:603–18.

Hagestad, Gunhild O. 1990. Social perspectives on the life course. In R. H. Binstock and L. K. George (eds.), *Handbook of Aging and the Social Sciences*, 3d ed. New York: Academic Press, pp. 151–68.

Havighurst, Robert J. 1963. Successful aging. In R. H. Williams et al. (eds.), *Processes of Aging: Social and Psychological Perspectives*. New York: Atherton, pp. 299–330.

James, William. 1890. *Principles of Psychology*. New York: Holt.

Johnson, Colleen L., and Barbara M. Barer. 1992. Patterns of disengagement among the oldest old. *Journal of Aging Studies* 6:351–64.

Kaufman, Sharon R. 1986. *The Ageless Self: Sources of Meaning in Later Life*. Madison, Wisc.: University of Wisconsin Press.

Kelly, George A. 1955. *The Psychology of Personal Constructs*. New York: Norton.

Kelly, John R. 1993. *Activity and Aging*. Newbury Park, Calif.: Sage.

Kinney, Jennifer M., M. A. P. Stephens, Melissa M. Franks, and V. K. Norris. 1995. Stresses and satisfactions of family caregivers to older stroke patients. *Journal of Applied Gerontology* 14:3–21.

Klapp, Orinn E. 1978. *Opening and Closing.* New York: Cambridge University Press.

Koenig, Harold G. 1995. *Aging and God.* New York: Haworth Pastoral Press.

Kogan, Nathan. 1990. Personality and aging. In J. E. Birren and K. W. Schaie (eds.), *Handbook of the Psychology of Aging,* 3d ed. New York: Academic Press, pp. 330–46.

Kunkel, Suzanne R., and Robert C. Atchley. 1996. Why gender matters: Being female is not the same as not being male. *American Journal of Preventive Medicine* 12:294–96.

Kuypers, Joseph A., and Vern L. Bengtson. 1973. Social breakdown and competence: A model of normal aging. *Human Development* 16:181–201.

Larson, Reed, Jiri Zuzanek, and Roger Mannell. 1985. Being alone versus being with people: Disengagement in the daily experience of older adults. *Journal of Gerontology* 40:375–81.

Lawton, M. Powell. 1975. The Philadelphia Geriatric Center Morale Scale: A revision. *Journal of Gerontology* 30:85–89.

Lemon, Bruce W., Vern L. Bengtson, and James A. Peterson. 1972. An exploration of the activity theory of aging: Activity types and life satisfaction among in-movers to a retirement community. *Journal of Gerontology* 27:511–23.

Levin, Jeffrey S. 1994. *Religion in Aging and Health.* Thousand Oaks, Calif.: Sage.

Levinson, Daniel J. 1978. *Seasons of a Man's Life.* New York: Knopf.

———. 1990. A theory of life structure development in adulthood. In C. N. Alexander and E. J. Langer (eds.), *Higher Stages of Human Development: Perspectives on Adult Growth.* New York: Oxford University Press, pp. 35–53.

Lieberman, Morton A., and Sheldon S. Tobin. 1983. *The Experience of Old Age: Stress, Coping, and Survival.* New York: Basic Books.

Longino, Charles F., Jr., and Cary S. Kart. 1982. Explicating activity theory: A formal replication. *Journal of Gerontology* 37:713–22.

Lopata, Helena Z. 1996. *Current Widowhood: Myths and Realities.* Thousand Oaks, Calif.: Sage.

Luborsky, Mark R. 1994. The cultural diversity of physical disability: The erosion of full personhood. *Journal of Aging Studies* 8:239–53.

Maddox, George L. 1968. Persistence of life style among the elderly: A longitudinal study of patterns of social activity in relation to life satisfaction. In B. L. Neugarten (ed.), *Middle Age and Aging.* Chicago: University of Chicago Press.

Maehr, Martin L., and Douglas A. Kleiber. 1981. The graying of achievement motivation. *American Psychologist* 36:787–93.

Mannell, Roger. 1993. High-investment activity and life satisfaction among older adults: Committed, serious leisure, and flow activities. In J. R. Kelly (ed.), *Activity and Aging.* Newbury Park, Calif.: Sage, pp. 125–45.

Markus, Hazel R., and A. Regula Herzog. 1991. The role of the self concept in aging. *Annual Review of Gerontology and Geriatrics* 11:110–43.

Markus, Hazel R., and Paula Nurius. 1986. Possible selves. *American Psychologist* 41:954–69.

McCrae, Robert R. 1995. Personality. In G. L. Maddox et al. (eds.), *Encyclopedia of Aging*, 2d ed. New York: Springer, pp. 735–36.

Miller, Stephen J. 1965. The social dilemma of the aging leisure participant. In A. M. Rose and W. A. Peterson (eds.), *Older People and Their Social World*. Philadelphia: Davis, pp. 77–92.

Morris, John N., and Sylvia Sherwood. 1975. A retesting and modification of the Philadelphia Geriatric Center Morale Scale. *Journal of Gerontology* 30:77–84.

Palmore, Erdman. 1964. Retirement patterns among aged men: Findings of the 1963 Survey of the Aged. *Social Security Bulletin* 27(6):3–10.

Parnes, Herbert S. 1981. *Work and Retirement: A Longitudinal Study of Men.* Cambridge, Mass.: MIT Press.

———. 1985. *Retirement among American Men.* Lexington, Mass.: D. C. Heath.

Pearlin, Leonard I. 1991. Life strains and psychological distress among adults. In A. Monat and R. S. Lazarus (eds.), *Stress and Coping: An Anthology*, 3d ed. New York: Columbia University Press, pp. 319–36.

Pollman, A. William. 1971. Early retirement: A comparison of poor health and other retirement factors. *Journal of Gerontology* 26:41–45.

Riegel, Klaus F. 1976. The dialectics of human development. *American Psychologist* 31:689–700.

Rodin, Judith, and Ellen Langer. 1977. Long-term effect of a control-relevant intervention. *Journal of Personality and Social Psychology* 36:12–29.

Roman, Paul, and Philip Taietz. 1967. Organizational structure and disengagement: The emeritus professor. *Gerontologist* 7:147–52.

Rosow, Irving. 1967. *Social Integration of the Aged.* New York: Free Press.

Ryff, Carol D. 1984. Personality development from the inside: The subjective experience of change in adulthood and aging. In P. B. Baltes and O. G. Brim, Jr. (eds.), *Life-Span Development and Behavior*, vol. 6. New York: Academic Press, pp. 243–79.

Selltiz, Claire, Marie Jahoda, Morton Deutch, and Stuart A. Cook. 1962. *Research Methods in Social Relations.* New York: Holt, Rinehart, and Winston.

Sill, John Stewart. 1980. Disengagement reconsidered: Awareness of finitude. *Gerontologist* 20:457–62.

Simpson, Ida H., and John C. McKinney (eds.). 1966. *Social Aspects of Aging.* Durham, N.C.: Duke University Press.

Skaff, Marilyn M. 1995. Stress and coping. In G. L. Maddox et al. (eds.) *Encyclopedia of Aging*, 2d ed. New York: Springer, pp. 900–902.

Streib, Gordon F., and Clement J. Schneider. 1971. *Retirement in American Society.* Ithaca, N.Y.: Cornell University Press.

Tornstam, Lars. 1994. Gero-transcendence: A theoretical and empirical exploration.

In L. E. Thomas and S. A. Eisenhandler (eds.), *Aging and the Religious Dimension.* Westport, Conn.: Auburn House, pp. 203–29.

Troll, Lillian E. 1982. *Continuations: Adult Development and Aging.* Monterey, Calif.: Brooks/Cole.

Verbrugge, Lois M., and Alan M. Jette. 1994. The disablement process. *Social Science and Medicine* 38:1–14.

Wesley, E. 1953. Preservative behavior in a concept-formation task as a function of manifest anxiety and rigidity. *Journal of Abnormal and Social Psychology* 48:129–34.

Wilber, Ken. 1996. *Eye to Eye,* 3d ed. Boston: Shambala.

Williams, Richard H., and Claudine Wirths. 1965. *Lives through the Years.* New York: Atherton.

Index

Achenbaum, Andrew W., 140
activities: continuity of, 3, 11, 20, 24–26,
57, 67–69, 74, 75, 77, 103, 104, 113,
115, 131, 150, 151; cutting back on, 67,
69, 70, 75, 101, 102, 107, 111, 119, 120,
125, 126; decline with continuity, 109–
10, 113, 114, 115, 116–17, 118, 149;
decline with offsets, 106, 108, 110–11,
113, 114, 116, 118, 120, 121, 122, 132,
151, 152; increases in, 67, 68, 69, 107,
109, 149; lifestyle, 10, 54, 67, 70–74,
118, 153; organizational, 19, 24, 54, 59,
61, 64, 65, 67–70, 72, 75, 107–11, 115,
119, 120, 123; physical, 54, 59, 67, 70,
71, 75; social, 48, 54, 59, 61, 69, 70, 71;
solitary, 54, 59, 61, 69–70, 72–73, 75;
substitution of new, 103, 104, 105, 106,
114, 115; trends in, 113–14, 116
Activities of Daily Living (ADLs), 16, 103,
115, 117, 118
activity frequencies, distribution of, 59–61
activity levels, 47, 50, 138; above average,
120, 126; and age, 57, 58, 59, 63–64, 74,
104, 105, 119; average, 122, 123, 125;
changes in, 31–32, 61–64, 89–91; continuity in overall, 61–70, 74–75, 85,
103–6, 113–15, 121, 150–52; and disability, xii, 93; and emotional resilience,
43–44; by employment status and gender, 88, 89; and gender and education,
52, 57–58; and health, 28, 57, 59, 63,
71, 72, 73, 74, 112, 120, 124, 129; and
morale, 26, 31, 90–93, 111, 112, 114,
115, 123, 124; negative changes in, 126,
129; patterns of, 62–63, 65–68, 113;
predictors of, 57–59, 63–65, 74, 128;

and retirement, 85, 88–89; and self-
confidence, 18, 25, 26, 37, 38, 41, 57, 58,
63, 74, 123, 124; and widowhood, 89,
123
activity patterns, 1, 4, 9, 103–26, 154, 158;
by activity type, 66; consolidation in,
103–7, 109, 113, 114, 115–16, 118; continuity of, 53–75, 103–5, 106, 113, 116,
151, 155; drastic changes in, 31–32
activity profiles, 1, 5, 75, 156
activity theory, ix, 1, 103, 104, 115, 117,
142
adaptation: of activity patterns, 103–26; to
aging, vii, ix, xi, xiii, 2, 7, 8, 13, 15, 16,
53, 76–77, 99, 116, 118, 147; to change,
vii, viii, ix, xiii, 1, 2, 7, 72, 76–78, 131;
and continuity, xiii, 6, 8, 79, 129, 131,
132, 153, 154; and continuity theory, 5–
9, 76–79, 91, 99, 102, 103, 105, 113,
116, 153; to disability, 20, 103–7, 115,
131, 153; to functional limitations, 91–
93, 107–18; general patterns of, 118–
26; to retirement, ix–xii, 2, 14–15, 48,
77, 78, 87, 89, 91, 118–19, 131; to role
loss, vii, viii, 103, 115, 116, 153
adaptive capacity, 1, 6, 9, 11–12, 76–132;
definition of, 78
ADLs. See Activities of Daily Living
age, 39, 43, 52; and activity levels, 57, 58,
59, 63–64, 74, 104, 105, 119; and personal agency, 95, 96, 97, 99
age discrimination, x, 13, 105, 158
aging, viii, 48, 59, 155; adaptation to, vii,
ix, xi, xiii, 2, 7, 8, 13, 15, 16, 53, 76–77,
99, 116, 118, 147; and change, 2, 6, 132,
147; development vs., 1, 12–13; effects

aging (*cont.*)
  on self of, 96, 99, 101–2, 140; as gentle
  slope, 13–18, 24, 31, 37, 96, 101, 118–
  20, 121, 126, 129, 132, 139, 158; physical, 12, 33, 76, 140; psychological, 12,
  140; and self-confidence, 7, 13, 17, 24,
  37, 39, 118, 119, 120; social, 12–13,
  140–41, 145; and spiritual development,
  139–42, 158
Anderson, Barbara, 45
Atchley, Robert, 10, 34

beliefs, viii, 5, 9, 33, 34, 78, 80, 137; about
  retirement, 47–51, 160
Bengtson, Vern L., 10
Buckley, Walter, xi, 5

caregiving, vii, 23, 121, 122, 123, 124, 132,
  153
case studies, xiii, 13–32, 70–73, 106, 107–
  12, 118–26; Betty, 108–9; Cathy, 71;
  Charles, 111–12; Cynthia, 120–22, 152;
  Dale, 17–18; Dennis, 119–20; Dolores,
  26–30; Doris, 108; Dorothy, 72; Edna,
  18–20; Elaine, 24–26; Frances, 111;
  Giles, 21–24, 153; Gordon, 118–19;
  Gwen, 13–16; Jane, 30–32; Joanne,
  122–23; John, 72; June, 107; Kay, 70;
  Ken, 71–72; Lyle (carpenter), 72; Lyle
  (lawyer), 112; Lynn, 119–20; Martha,
  110; Matilda, 123–24; Mike, 24–26;
  Ned, 107; Patrick, 73; Roger, 122, 152,
  153; Ruth, 109–10; Sally, 119; Stella,
  125–26; Stephen, 71; Ted, 13–16; Tess,
  37; Thelma, 109; Vera, 110; Walter, 108;
  Wayne, 124–25, 152
change, 41, 80; in activity levels, 31–32,
  61–64, 89–91, 126, 129; adaptation to,
  vii, viii, ix, xiii, 1, 2, 7, 72, 76–78, 131;
  and aging, 2, 6, 132, 147; and continuity,
  2–3, 32, 74, 77, 85, 98, 99, 100, 101,
  102, 131–32, 133, 148, 150; coping
  with, vii, 76–78, 105, 124, 132, 154; in
  emotional resilience, 97–98, 101; and
  gender differences, 89, 127, 128, 129; in
  health, viii, 12, 15–16, 31, 52, 101, 120;
  in life course, 6, 8, 41; in lifestyle, 76,
  101, 118, 122, 126; in marital status, 55,
  56, 89–90; in morale, ix, 21, 86, 89–90,
  110–11, 127, 129; negative, 126–30; in
  patterns of activity, 31–32; in personal

goals, 97–98, 102, 134; substantial, 18–
  24, 118, 120–23; in values, 6, 15, 30, 45,
  80, 101
Chow test, 40
Clark, Margaret, 45
continuity: of activities, 3, 11, 20, 24–26,
  57, 67–69, 74, 75, 77, 103, 104, 113,
  115, 131, 150, 151; in activity levels, 61–
  70, 74–75, 85, 103–6, 113–15, 121,
  150–52; of activity patterns, 53–75,
  103–5, 106, 113, 116, 151, 155; and
  adaptation, xiii, 6, 8, 79, 129, 131, 132,
  153, 154; and change, 2–3, 32, 74, 77,
  85, 98, 99, 100, 101, 102, 131–32, 133,
  148, 150; of community, 74; and coping,
  xiii, 12, 24, 76–78, 79, 80, 82, 84, 147,
  154; definition of, 4, 8, 148, 157; desire
  for, 8, 130, 131, 133, 136–39; of dwelling, 56, 71, 74; in emotional resilience,
  43, 44, 51, 99, 102, 131, 152; evolutionary forms of, 151, 157; external, 9, 10–
  11, 53–75, 77, 78, 84, 85, 131, 133, 151,
  154; as feedback systems theory, 5, 150,
  157; and frameworks of ideas, 33, 151,
  152, 154, 155, 158; and health, 23, 78,
  85, 138, 152; in household composition,
  xiii, 55, 56, 74; in income adequacy, 54,
  56, 78, 85, 131, 135; internal, 9–10, 33–
  52, 77, 78, 84, 85, 88, 131, 133, 151,
  154; and life satisfaction, 7, 54, 150, 154,
  155, 158; in lifestyles, xiii, 2, 13, 20, 24,
  53–54, 56, 57, 73, 74, 130–32, 135–38,
  146, 150, 152; and longitudinal patterns,
  4, 152; measurement of, 3, 4, 36, 62; of
  mental constructs, 9, 52, 151, 155, 156;
  of morale, 13, 85, 114, 116, 127–28,
  154; orientation toward, 79–80; patterns
  of, 61, 62, 64, 65, 68, 151, 158; of personal agency, 10, 95, 96, 101–2, 151,
  152–53; in personal goals, xiii, 2, 5, 34,
  46, 51, 97–98, 99, 101, 133–36, 138,
  150, 152, 154, 156, 157; and positive
  attitudes, 12, 16, 17; predisposition toward, xiii, 18, 26, 136–39; prevalence of,
  148, 149, 150, 151; of relationships, 11,
  16, 131, 137, 150; in retirement beliefs,
  50, 51; of the self, 10, 34, 100, 102, 118;
  of self-confidence, xiii, 16, 17, 24, 39,
  41, 51, 152; and spiritual development,
  141, 145; and stability, 3, 36, 52, 68, 98,
  148, 151; strategies for, 7, 24, 154–55;

unadulterated, 13–18, 99; in values, 14, 102, 131, 138, 150

continuity theory, vii, viii, 1–32, 93, 95; and adaptation, 6, 7, 8–9, 76, 77, 78, 79, 91, 99, 102, 103, 105, 113, 116, 153; applications of, 157–58; assessing, 148–55; assumptions of, 8, 9, 148, 150, 151–52, 154, 155; development of, xiii, 1–7; elements of, 9–12; and future research, xiii, 147, 156–58; identity in, x, xii; and methodological issues, 155–56; on personality and temperament, 33, 156; propositions of, 8, 9, 148, 150, 152–54, 155; as theory, 1, 4–9

coping, 9, 13, 23, 42; with activity loss, 102–7; with aging, 77, 121, 147; with change, vii, 76–78, 105, 124, 132, 154; and continuity, xiii, 12, 24, 76–78, 79, 80, 82, 84, 147, 154; definition of, 76; with functional limitations, 91–93, 107–18, 153; and marriage, 12, 16, 17, 18; proactive, xiii, 78–79, 82, 131; reactive, 131; and religion, 12, 20, 26, 30, 32, 82, 83, 84, 120, 122, 126, 131; with retirement, xiii, 16, 18, 85–89, 125; and social support networks, 26, 122, 124, 126, 131; strategies for, 76, 78, 80, 82–85, 114, 123, 131, 148; with widowhood, 89–91. *See also* adaptation

Cumming, Elaine, ix

death, 143; fear of, 20, 32, 119, 142, 144, 145, 154; meaning of, 139, 141; and retirement, 48

decision making, ix, 7, 152, 153, 156

depression. *See* morale

development, adult: and adaptive capacity, 77–78; aging *vs.*, 1, 12–13; and child development, xii, 2; continuous, xi–xii; and feedback systems theory, 4–5; goals for direction in, xiii, 5–6, 11, 78, 133–46; spiritual, xiii, 11, 133, 139–42, 145–46, 154, 157, 158; stages of, vii, viii, 33

disability, xii, xiii, 2, 13, 41, 93–107; adaptation to, 20, 103–7, 115, 131, 153; and continuity strategies, 7, 24; definition of functional, 97; and emotional resilience, 93, 94, 99, 100, 102; extreme, 12, 52, 77, 102, 132; increasing, 28, 29; onset of, 91–93; patterns of coping with, 107–18; and personal agency, 93–94, 95, 96, 99;

100, 101, 112, 116, 131; and personal goals, 94, 100; and scale scores, 97, 106; and the self, 93–107; studies of, 102–3. *See also* functional limitations

discontinuity, viii, 23; continuity *vs.*, xii, xiii, 155; and disability, 13, 30, 130; of dwelling, 25–26; measurement of, 64; and morale, 9, 132, 154–55; patterns of, 3, 4, 36, 37, 61, 64–65, 68, 134, 148, 149; and personal goals, 46, 99; unwanted, 24–32, 123–26, 155

disengagement, ix, 105, 106, 132; and functional limitation, 103, 104, 111–12, 113, 114, 115, 117, 153

disengagement theory, ix, 105, 117, 142

Duke Longitudinal Study, 1

education, xiii, 40, 43, 71; and activity level, 52, 58, 63; and personal agency, 95, 96, 97, 99

emotional resilience, 34, 41–44, 52, 94, 159; analysis of scores, 42–44; change in, 97–98, 101; continuity in, 43, 44, 51, 99, 102, 131, 152; and disability, 93, 94, 99, 100, 102; predictors of, 44; and self, 101–2

employment, 17, 46, 54, 87, 88, 89; and work identity, ix, x, 1–2, 14, 24

equilibrium, 1, 103, 117, 151; maintenance of activity, 104, 106, 113, 115, 116. *See also* activity theory

Erikson, Erik H., xii

feedback systems theory, xi, 4, 5, 7, 150, 157

functional capability, 28, 31, 43, 52, 63, 81, 152; loss of, 77, 78, 85, 91–93, 126, 130; and self-confidence, 37, 38, 39–40, 41

functional limitations, 121, 131–32, 152, 155; and activity patterns, 112–13; and chronic conditions, 102–3, 106; and disengagement, 103, 104, 111–12, 113, 114, 115, 117, 153; patterns of coping with, 91–93, 107–18, 153; and the self, 93–106. *See also* disability

gender, x, xiii, 40, 43, 84; and activity level, 52, 57–58, 59, 63, 88, 89; and change, 89, 127, 128, 129; and personal agency, 95, 96, 97, 99

gerontology, vii–xii, 1, 52, 103, 142

gerotranscendence, 119, 133, 141–42, 144–45, 154
gerotranscendence theory, 142–45, 157
Guttman scale, 106

health: and activity levels, 28, 57, 59, 63, 71–74, 112, 120, 124, 129; changes in, viii, 12, 15–16, 31, 52, 101, 120; concerns about, 13, 14, 15, 22, 27, 28; and continuity, 23, 78, 85, 138, 152; and preventive practices, 17, 18, 19, 21, 24, 30–31, 80–81, 82, 119, 120, 122; and retirement, 13–17, 22–23, 24–25, 27, 48, 118, 119, 122; and self-confidence, 19, 37, 38, 41; self-rated, 38, 43, 44, 52, 57, 58, 63, 81, 124, 126, 128, 129, 132, 149–50, 152
Henry, William, ix
Herzog, A. Regula, 10, 37, 102
hobbies: continuity in, 23, 65, 69; and lifestyles, 54, 59, 61, 69, 70, 72, 73, 74, 75; participation in, 61, 67, 71, 111, 112, 120, 121. See also activities; lifestyles
homemakers, full-time, 70, 111, 122; status of, 26–27
household composition, xiii, 54–55, 56, 74

IADL. See Instrumental Activities of Daily Living
identity continuity theory, x, xii
identity crisis theory, x
income adequacy, viii, ix; continuity in, 54, 56, 78, 85, 131, 135
Instrumental Activities of Daily Living (IADL), 115
Internet, 121–22, 152

Kaufman, Sharon R., 134
Kelly, George, xii
Koenig, Harold G., 83

Langer, Ellen, 10
Levinson, Daniel J., 5n
life course, vii, xi, 6, 8, 41, 152, 153
life rating, 132, 152; predictors of, 128, 129
life satisfaction, 11, 118, 122, 145, 152; and continuity, 7, 54, 150, 154, 155, 158
lifestyles, viii, 5, 6, 9, 10–11; and adaptation to aging, vii, 7, 8, 13, 15, 16, 53, 118, 147; changes in, 76, 101, 118, 122,

126; continuity in, xiii, 2, 13, 20, 24, 53–54, 56, 57, 73, 74, 130–32, 135–38, 145, 150, 152; diversified, 70–71, 73, 75; and hobbies, 54, 59, 61, 69, 70, 72, 73, 74, 75; and household composition, xiii, 54–55, 56, 74; and marital status, 54, 55, 56; minimal involvement, 70, 73–74, 75; and organizational participation, 61, 72, 73; and patterns of activities, xiii, 1, 9, 11, 153; and physical activity, 59, 71–72, 73; and socializing, 23, 59, 61, 64, 65, 68, 71, 73, 75, 123; and social roles, 9, 10, 77, 91; and solitary activities, 54, 59, 61, 69–70, 72–73, 75; and volunteer service, 14, 15, 16, 54. See also activities; living arrangements; relationships
living arrangements, xiii, 9, 10, 31, 54–56; continuity in, 1, 131, 135, 149, 150; and personal goals, 134; by residential mobility status, 55

Maddox, George, 1
Markus, Hazel R., 10, 37, 102
marriage: and coping, 12, 16, 17, 18; and moving, 55–56; relationships in, 14–18, 21, 23, 24, 25, 27, 28, 70–71, 72; and remarriage, 91, 131; and retirement, 118, 120; satisfaction with, 121, 122, 123
measurement of continuity, 3, 4; external continuity, 62; inner continuity, 36
mental frameworks, 4–5, 6, 7, 147
morale, ix, 2, 16, 20, 75; and activity level, 26, 31, 90–93, 111, 112, 114, 115, 123, 124; and aging, 17, 24, 145; average, 22, 24, 73, 109, 110, 111, 121, 122, 126; change in, ix, 21, 86, 89–90, 110–11, 127, 129; continuity of, 13, 85, 114, 116, 127–28, 154; and discontinuity, 8, 9, 132, 154–55; and disposition toward continuity, 138; and functional ability, 92, 144, 154; high, 27, 28, 30, 31, 107, 108, 110, 118, 119, 120, 123; and illness, 23, 24, 122; predictors of, 128–30; reduced, 21, 25, 26, 29, 115, 116, 125, 126, 152; and retirement, 15, 17, 19, 85–88, 89; scale of, 4, 41–42; stability in, 107–8; trend in, 113–14; and widowhood, 89–90, 91, 123

National Institute of Mental Health, xi
National Longitudinal Studies of the

Labor Market Experiences of Mature Men, xi
Normative Aging Study, xi
Nurius, Paula, 10
nursing homes, 8, 54, 55

Ohio Longitudinal Study of Aging and Adaptation (OLSAA), 85, 107, 118, 161–71; beginning of, x, xii, 13, 24; continuity and discontinuity in, 149; and continuity theory, 34, 137, 154, 156; descriptive analyses of, 35–37, 42–43, 45–46, 48–50, 89–93; funding of, xi; and future research, 147–48; inventory of personal goals, 134, 140; multivariate analyses of, 37–41, 43–44, 46–47, 50; path analysis of, 93–94, 95; and patterns of activity, 59, 67, 69; regression analyses of, 38–41, 52, 57, 58, 59, 63–70, 74, 81, 94, 129, 151, 156; and research on gerotranscendence, 143–45; survey of lifestyles in, 54, 57, 59
Ohio Long-Term Care Research Project, xi
OLSAA. *See* Ohio Longitudinal Study of Aging and Adaptation
Orwoll, Lucinda, 140

Pearlin, Leonard I., 77
personal agency, 33–34, 37, 111; continuity of, 10, 95, 96, 101–2, 151, 152–53; data on, 94, 98, 137; and functional disability, 93–94, 95, 96, 99, 100, 101, 112, 116, 131
personal constructs, 6, 9, 77, 151, 158
personal construct theory, xii
personal goals, 9, 11, 12, 14, 27, 44–49, 52, 160; and activity levels, 47, 63; and change, 97–98, 102, 134; continuity in, xiii, 2, 5, 34, 46, 51, 97–98, 99, 101, 133–36, 138, 150, 152, 154, 156, 157; and functional disability, 93, 95, 100, 102, 131; importance of, 45–46, 94; patterns of, 134–35; predictors of, 47, 48, 49; and self, 101–2, 140; and stability, 46, 47, 134; structure of, 151
Philadelphia Geriatric Center (PGC) Morale Scale, 4, 41–42

relationships, vii, 6, 7, 9, 10, 76, 82; continuity of, 11, 16, 131, 137, 150; family, viii, 11, 12, 14, 21, 27, 61, 112, 134, 135,
158; patterns of, 154, 155, 158; social, 1, 2, 31, 48, 150. *See also* marriage
religion, 2, 16, 21, 134, 135, 139, 157; and church attendance, 17, 30, 59, 61, 64, 65, 68–70, 75, 101, 108–10, 112, 120, 124; and coping, 12, 20, 26, 30, 32, 82, 83, 84, 120, 122, 126, 131; and gerotranscendence, 142–45. *See also* development, adult: spiritual; transcendence
research, vii–xii; future, xiii, 147–48, 150, 156–58; on gerotranscendence, 143–45; on retirement adaptation, ix–xii
retirement, viii, xiii; adaptation to, ix–xii, 2, 14–15, 48, 77, 78, 87, 91, 118–19, 131; attitudes toward, 13–19, 21, 22, 24–27, 30, 34, 109, 119–26, 128, 152; beliefs about, 47–51, 160; and continuity, 85, 135, 151, 152; and health, 13, 14, 15, 16, 17, 22–23, 24–25, 27, 48, 118, 119, 122; and morale, 15, 17, 19, 85–88, 89; planning for, 18–19; research on, ix–xii; and self-concepts, ix; and self-confidence, 17, 41; sources of income in, viii, ix
retirement communities, 31, 32, 54–55
Riegel, Klaus, xi
Rodin, Judith, 10

self, 5, 6; acceptance of, 45, 134, 135, 140, 146; and aging, 96, 99, 101–2, 140; continuity of, 10, 34, 100, 102, 118; and functional disability, 93–107; ideal, 9, 10; ideas about, 10, 33, 150; and life changes, 8, 133
self-concept, ix, 9, 10, 11, 14, 15, 34, 111; development of, 13, 150, 152, 153
self-confidence, xii, 23, 34, 35–41, 52; and activity levels, 18, 25, 26, 37, 38, 41, 57, 58, 63, 74, 123, 124; and aging, 7, 13, 17, 24, 37, 39, 118, 119, 120; average, 24, 122, 126; continuity in, xiii, 16, 17, 24, 39, 41, 51, 152; decline in, 36, 122, 123, 124, 125, 126, 153, 155; and functional capability, 37, 39–40; and health, 19, 37, 38, 41; high, 24, 27, 30, 31, 39, 58, 121, 123; increase in, 36; lowering of, 21, 22, 25, 26, 28, 29, 132; predictors of, 37, 38, 39, 40, 41, 128–29
self-esteem, ix, x, 7, 10
self-reliance, 15, 45, 134, 135, 141
self-striving, 10, 11. *See also* personal goals

self-values, 10, 99. *See also* personal goals
social class, xiii, 11
social isolation, vii, ix, 30
social opportunities, 53, 105
Social Security, ix, 73, 108
social support networks, ix, 5, 11, 16, 20, 128; and aging, 13, 77; continuity in, 15, 78, 123; and coping, 26, 122, 124, 126, 131
stability, viii, xii, 4, 53–54, 57, 88; and continuity, 3, 36, 52, 68, 98, 148, 151; in morale, 107–8; patterns of, 64, 65; and personal goals, 46, 47, 134
stage theories, xii

theories, ix–xii; activity, ix, 1, 103, 104, 115, 117, 142; disengagement, ix, 105, 117, 142; feedback systems, xi, 4, 5, 7, 150, 157; gerotranscendence, 142–45, 157; identity continuity, x, xii; identity crisis, x; personal construct, xii; stage, xii. *See also* continuity theory
Tornstam, Lars, 142–44
transcendence, 10, 12, 33, 139, 140, 157. *See also* gerotranscendence
transportation, 54, 57, 74

values, viii, ix, 9, 33, 78, 134, 136; and change, 6, 15, 30, 45, 80, 101; continuity in, 14, 102, 131, 138, 150; religious, 2, 101; self, 10, 99
volunteer service, 14, 15, 16, 54, 120

well-being, subjective, 103, 105, 106, 115, 116, 117; and activity loss, 104, 107, 112
Wesley, E., 80
Wesley Mental Rigidity Inventory, 80
widowhood, viii, xiii, 18, 29, 149; adaptation to, 77, 78, 123, 131; and continuity, 2, 13, 85, 152; and lifestyle, 55, 56, 72; and morale, 89–90, 91, 123; and self-confidence, 41, 123
Wilber, Ken, 10
Williams, Richard H., 7
Wirths, Claudine, 7
wisdom, 12, 139, 140, 142, 144, 158
women, ix, x, xiii, 56, 84, 87, 88; and activity levels, 52, 59. *See also* gender; widowhood
work identity, ix, x, 1–2, 14, 24

About the Author

Robert C. Atchley received a B.A. from Miami University and a Ph.D. in sociology from American University. He joined the faculty of Miami University, in Oxford, Ohio, in 1966. From 1974 to 1998 he was director of the Scripps Gerontology Center there. In 1984 he was named distinguished professor of gerontology in the Department of Sociology, Gerontology, and Anthropology. He is currently professor and chair of the Department of Gerontology at the Naropa Institute, in Boulder, Colorado. His gerontology research interests include adult development, spiritual development, long-term care, public policy, work and retirement, health change and disability, and family issues.

Dr. Atchley is the author of more than 85 journal articles and book chapters in the social science literature on aging and more than a dozen books and research monographs, including *The Sociology of Retirement* (1976), *Aging: Continuity and Change* (1987), and eight editions of his introductory text *Social Forces and Aging* (1997). He is associate editor of *The Encyclopedia of Aging* and was founding editor of *Contemporary Gerontology: A Journal of Reviews and Critical Discourse.*

Dr. Atchley was president of the American Society on Aging from 1988 to 1990 and has served in numerous leadership roles in the Gerontological Society of America, the American Society on Aging, and the Association for Gerontology in Higher Education. He has received more than a dozen awards for his scholarship, teaching, and service in the field of aging.

Library of Congress Cataloging-in-Publication Data

Atchley, Robert C.
   Continuity and adaptation in aging : creating positive
experiences / Robert C. Atchley.
      p.   cm.
   Includes index.
   ISBN 0-8018-6122-5 (alk. paper)
   1. Adjustment (Psychology) in old age — Longitudinal studies.
2. Happiness in old age — Longitudinal studies.   I. Title.
BF724.8.A8   1999
155.67′2 — dc21   98-51019
                                        CIP